HONOUR YOUR POSTPARTUM

Honour Your Postpartum

THE POSTPARTUM IS FOR EVERY WOMB THAT HAS CARRIED LIFE™

Naomie Karemi KAINGU

Contents

DEDICATION	ix
ACKNOWLEDGEMENTS	xi
She arrived home...	xv

One
BIRTH IS A CEREMONY — 1

Two
THE ANCESTRAL POSTPARTUM PERIOD — 6

Three
FIRST THEY WERE UNVEILED — 17

Four
THEN THEY WERE WELCOMED AND HONOURED — 24

Five
FINALLY THEY WERE CLOSED AND CELEBRATED — 28

Six
SUPPORT STARTS FROM WITHIN — 34

Seven
SUPPORT COMES FROM PEOPLE WHO SEE YOUR NEED — 42

Eight
WHEN YOU VISIT... — 47

Nine
IF IT DOES NOT SOUND RIGHT, DO NOT SAY IT 64

Ten
EMPTY HANDS, FULL BREASTS 69

Eleven
HONOUR YOUR POSTPARTUM 75

Twelve
HONOR YOUR POSTPARTUM - SPLIT 79

Thirteen
CELEBRATE YOUR PROGRESS 96

Fourteen
THRIVE...DON'T SURVIVE 107

Fifteen
IMPERFECTLY PERFECT 112

Sixteen
YOUR OTHER/OLDER CHILDREN 115

Seventeen
THE SNAP-BACK MENTALITY 121

Eighteen
YOUR CARE PROVIDERS 127

Nineteen
QUESTIONS TO ASK YOUR CARE PROVIDERS 132

Twenty
FROM ONE PARENT TO ANOTHER - TIPS 135

Twenty-One
POSTPARTUM STORIES SHARED WITH ME 141

Twenty-Two
HOMEMADE RECIPES TO TRY 152

About The Author 162

DEDICATION

This is for my maternal grandmother, **NYEVU**.

She taught me so much as a young girl, and she continues to pour into me every time I get to spend time with her. Her wisdom I will carry through generations. Her resilience is one I admire, and her selfless personality makes her my own Princess Diana, as I call her.

In Swahili, we call grandmothers '**Nyanya**'. My Nyanya Nyevu has been the force, encouragement, and engine behind this book and my work as an Ancestral Birth worker & trainer. She poured into me something that I had never heard before. Many say they had not even read in books that I have shared the wisdom with. Nyanya Nyevu practiced as a traditional MKUNGA (Birth worker) in her community, having learned the RITES and ways from her mother.

She helped birth many of my cousins.

I am in awe at her calm, her knowledge, and wisdom through ALL the RITES of passages I have encountered with her

My mother, **JOSEPHINE KIBIBI,** preserved the **RITES** and culture of our people. Her teachings and guidance throughout my life have been in line with the ways of our people. She encourages me to understand, seek, and preserve the rituals for generations to come. She instills wisdom in me to date.

My mother encouraged me to speak to the 'horse' (my grandmother) directly, which I did in 2020, and filmed her. I could ask questions I had, so that I got the real juice from Nyanya Nyevu. As the next in line, I promise to preach about this work, the Mijikenda, as an example of how beautiful and profound our ways really are

ACKNOWLEDGEMENTS

Thank you to my husband, Tom, for always being my number one cheerleader in this work and path as I focused on my passion for highlighting this work because it is a gap. For all the family dinners he had to do in my absence with our children, the outings he took them so I could have alone timed to focus on this book, and all his encouragement throughout. Some days were hard, some evenings harder with little sleep, but he still held it together so I could focus on this production. Thank you, Tom. I love you.

My 11-year-old entertained her brothers many times when mama had to finish a chapter or when mama had to concentrate on the other brother. Lucia, I love you too. Alexander is my middle child living with a disability and sometimes just looking at him whenever I could I would whisper 'thank you too for being so adaptable with babysitters who came and went until we found a stable Nanny, Lavinia who enabled me to put my focus in this book. It would never have been easy like they all made it to be.

My mother, Josephine Kibibi, also lifted me up a lot. After the death of my father in January 2022, I lost track whilst grieving his death, and many times, she would remind me to try when I could. To know that my late father would have wanted me to continue. He always was encouraging to me, always blessing me and I know as a daughter, without fail I did the best by him. Thank you, mama

Many people would probably ask; why now? Well... I wanted to write about the ways, and the RITES of my people before anybody else did, who was not from it nor linked with the information directly because that would not have been me! I want to iterate the importance of mindfulness when we step foot into the spaces of birth and especially the postpartum period for the spiritual values that many are not in tune nor intuitive about

I wanted to press on the importance of why the Fourth Trimester is vital regardless of whether a baby lived, regardless of how long a pregnancy existed, from my Kenyan cultural perspective and why the focus within the (boma) homestead is the woman (she/her)

Copyright © 2022 by Naomie Karemi KAINGU
All rights reserved.
No portion of this book may be reproduced in any form without written permission from the publisher or author except as permitted by U.S. copyright law.

She arrived home...

But has she landed?

When visiting new parents, we often forget that things have not settled yet, mentally and spiritually. We overlook the spiritual aspects concerning birth and the vital adjustments in these fragile moments because the focus remains on the bump, not the moments after. When we step foot into the space of a postpartum family, we need to know that many clouds exist within that home.

It does not have to be sad because not all pregnancies are of misery and pain, but a 'void' is present in the first few weeks a family welcomes a new baby. Life as we know it is not a bed of roses, and being healthy is not a given. Birth is hard work, and recuperating is vital.

For many, there may be struggles and 'layers within. In my native country, Kenya, we say that a child born within the family is a returning ancestor. When the returning ancestor returns, there needs to be a moment to adjust within the community, and therefore, connections within the community are revived again. Hence our hold on family names.

Childbirth is not just a union where the family members meet. It is a reunion where ancestors make connections and family members make amends and aim for new beginnings.

The passing of family names signifies the continuing of a lineage. Spiritually, in these fragile moments, many doors are still open, and moments are still raw.

Being mindful of the energy we bring with us is essential. I sing about it everywhere I am given the opportunity to. As birth workers, knowing and understanding the essence of holding space and providing support beforehand can change how we support families and how they feel embraced or 'held' through the adjustments in this life-changing phase of anyone's life. *I wrote this book for everyone's encouragement and from my own observed need for the narrative to be changed.*

For the mothers to be honored and the sacredness of birth to be **RE-CLAIMED**. Birth is a journey that can remain open for a long time.

The westernized or current times of 6-8 weeks postpartum and the idea that a woman or birthing person is ok after the 8th week is where the problem starts. During the postpartum appointment, most of the topic is contraception and when you can conceive again. This book came about from my walks as a Doula, both in the Birth, postpartum, and bereavement phases.

I have witnessed people unaware of the sacredness of these raw spaces. Many are unaware of how mindful they should be in these sacred spaces. They are not aware of the weight of their words in this immediate yet fragile phase. I share my ancestral wisdom and am very humbled that this wisdom has landed in your hands, too.

Thank you for your support and willingness to change the narrative. In this book, I have used a combination of Woman, WombMan, she/her, and they to cover everyone. I associate as a woman (She/Her), and so does my mother. I am learning to use inclusive language, though please bear with me.

One

BIRTH IS A CEREMONY

And the postpartum period is a RITE of passage. A **RITE of passage** is the transition from childhood into adulthood, passing the different milestones like birth, puberty, adulthood, marriage, childbirth, and so forth.

Birth is a ceremony because a blessed womb is not a given. This RITE of passage demands we come together as a people to honor the life that has come forth and honor the womb that bore, nurtured, and then birthed the baby. Birth is a ceremony because the event brings people together in unity and celebration to welcome the return of a descendant or ancestor.

Birth is a ceremony; hence, communities availed themselves to the new parents without measure following the news of the birth of a baby. There is ancestral wisdom in the understanding of the moments following the birth of a baby. Ancestrally, the immediate and the first six weeks following the birth warrant that the birthing person does nothing. The birthing person with her family needs to recover and recuperate, and they cannot do that alone. It takes a village to help them do so.

Birth as a **RITE** of passage. It represents the growing up of a child into a parent and, therefore, an increment of a lineage. Though a **RITE** of passage, birth can be lonely and isolating. It is lonely because the mental load before the baby's birth and afterward enlarges regardless of how the birth took place.

As she births her baby (She/Her), the community comes together to offer support so that the newborn mother or person can connect with their baby and come back to their soul. She may use voice, whimper, pray and sing to welcome her baby. Many times, the people within the Manyatta would sing a tribal song or hum a song together to encourage her to focus and give her strength. The birth was a communal thing, and there was an understanding that there was a need for cheer. Otherwise, everyone followed the lead of the birthing person. But they did not leave her to wander with her thoughts.

They encouraged her to move and feel her body go through the change, clinging to support whenever she needed it or staying in her bubble while communicating with her baby in utero. Many songs sung in a birthing space or hummed were songs of the ancestors, what has happened within the tribe and what they look forward to achieving with the returning ancestor. It is usually a spiritually warming space, and the surrounding it understands the amount of spiritual strength and energy needed and used until the baby is born.

> **A lot of grief comes with the birth of a baby, too.**

An aspect that is never discussed or mentioned, even during the 'bump phase. At childbirth, a shift of energies, emotions, and personalities has to happen for one to grow. That shift brings sadness because it takes away a part of the person and replaces it with another they have to identify with so fast.

With every change, change and regrouping are necessary.

You will enter a space and exchange energy with your initial self, knowing very well that it is an event. You will come into the sphere of life and death, and then a **new you** will emerge, with a newborn baby whom you will learn to love and nurture in the outside world, with no manual to guide you other than advice from those near you and your maternal instincts. This shift is clear in a birthing room where the woman is in a daze. They hear and respond, but what they say sometimes makes little sense, showing signs they may not be 'with it.

That alone is a **load**! *When a baby is born, the mother is also born.* Therefore, the ceremony is aimed at lifting the newborn mother or parent and celebrating their victory because childbirth is like a battle. Few survive it, even though it IS a passage.

In the western world, everyone is busy working long hours to sustain their families. It is even more daunting. In many countries, new parents are sent home without instruction or guidance. They were often asked 'to call if there is a problem, knowing very well they are unlikely to reach out because the busyness that follows the moments they arrive home does not leave space to ask for guidance unless it is an emergency. So even when people surround you, you will find their journeys and understanding different from yours.

Some parents birth babies with special needs, and others birth babies who have different capabilities and needs. So even amongst families, you cannot compare the experience from one to another. So while we search for the 'village' in the western world, many still cry behind closed doors, not knowing how or where to look for the village amongst them to belong. Even when others surround you, the loneliness is profound.

The wisdom that birth and the postpartum period are milestones is still not understood. Unfortunately, for many, where generations have changed ways, wisdom is being forgotten and almost becoming extinct. It is frowned upon as 'old wives' tales' in many areas or deemed backward.

As a developed society in these times, looking after mothers or newborn parents is quickly done. Everyone deals with life their way, and families are scattered or disconnected. It is sad because if there was ever a moment that a person needed people around them; it was during the birth of a baby. This moment demands time, which is why, ancestrally, the outside world stayed away to give the new parents space to 'land' and come to be in their new roles as parents. The birthing mother (she/her) provides light, and the new father receives it and gives it back, forming the circle of love. That can only happen without disruptions.

There was also a reason, ancestrally, people gathered around to support. Some people find the isolation ok and are happy to continue by themselves, but that is not how this moment is supposed to be. It is hard work to carry, nurture, and then birth a baby. It is hard to figure out what to do in those first few hours following the birth of a baby, especially when you have to show up for others in that same bubble.

And in all honesty, we were never meant to go through this phase of the passages alone. People traveled far and near to avail themselves of where the baby was born because it was understood that food, nurturing, and others were vital at this moment. The birth of a baby in any lineage means that the family lineage is being extended. The birth of the baby means an ancestor has returned. Where there were woes, disagreements, or unresolved issues within a community, the birth of a baby symbolizes a new beginning for everyone within the clan or tribe.

They prioritized both mother and baby in the clan because they remained in the gateways of life and death. The focus to fend, feed, nurture, and then protect lies with the elders and the extended lineage within the clan. Therefore, those 'concerned' would ensure the homestead is protected because the mother and child are not in danger immediately after childbirth.

In your postpartum bed, you are still bleeding, and the placenta wound in your womb is very open. Your energy is deficient, your mental health is foggy or clouded, and your head is running fast with everything you need to remember. You will need to suddenly learn (because nobody is born a mother!), and your spiritual energy or antenna is very open. You are, therefore, very receptive to energies and influences, too.

Do I have a tip for family and friends? Of course! :-)

The moments after childbirth are moments to allow your loved ones this time to bond and enjoy their 'hello bubble. Disrupting this bubble is doing them an injustice as a family. Let them be for now. Cook and deliver the meals without going into the bedroom to have a peep or disrupt their calm. She is still bleeding, probably not in the mood yet to have the entire clan around because giving birth is prominent, and she needs time to recover. Wait for their say and welcome before showing up, even if you were next door visiting the neighbor.

Remember: Just because they were sent home from the hospital does not mean they came home (yet). Let them 'arrive' and find each other first. With childbirth, some detachment happens between the new parents because they see each other differently.

Two

THE ANCESTRAL POSTPARTUM PERIOD

In the immediate postpartum (day one to three), your body is naturally in shock. You may be startled, trying to make sense of what happened. You would find many newborn mothers are still high on adrenaline and maybe even still not with it. Many are astonished they could achieve the births they had planned for and simply could not switch their minds off.

Many parents say it either felt like they could not get down from 'the high' and it exhausted them in the long run. Others share it felt like a cloud had set in, demanding that they stayed in the 'now' but 'still functioned. It is wise to be mindful of the space in this mode, especially for the birthing partner, who is more conscious at this moment. Be mindful of being in this mode (being on a high) for far too long. It could exhaust you in the long run. Speak with someone you trust about your birth experience. Speak about what you imagined it would be like and what it was like so that you can find a place for your experience, to open up for more that is to come, because parenthood is a long journey.

The difference between the old ways and the modern times of a postpartum is that **the daze and confusion** are often missed and the birthing person is left searching and yearning within themselves to connect the pieces of the puzzle. Even with the modernized way of living where moments are captured on phones, the puzzles never seem to make sense because the important parts are missed out. The part where the birthing person is embraced and cared for in love and gentleness. Where she may be in the moment without the pressure of checking things, where she is nurtured in her most confused state and also celebrated.

The haze or still moment is part of the reason all the attention in the immediate postpartum just after childbirth was aimed at the birthing person because there is a significant shift that happens that demands attention. Because this is the moment of 'nothingness' where the birthing person is only pampered and looked after ceremonially, it is a moment to refuel because once everyone who availed themselves went back to their lives, the parenting duty really begins.

Compare the statement above with the modern Postpartum, where a maternity nurse who acts as the intermediate between the hospital and the midwife comes to you every day for the first eight or ten days (typically in the Netherlands) or in a country like the UK where a health visitor comes to see you at home a few times every week or every other week before the sixth-week appointment where you are invited to go back for your six-week check-up before your medical file is closed.

In the case of the Maternity nurses in the Netherlands, what I see as a Maternity nurse myself is that the list of advice and information is so overwhelming that as an Ancestral birth worker, I trade carefully. I work understanding that many times the first 4 days, a newborn mother needs time to bring the pieces of the puzzle together and 'land' that adding a whole list or booklet of information to them adds a whole new load to their already overloaded mental load which is unnecessary (yet)

If we go with a typical maternity nurse available to your family for the 8 days as standard in the Netherlands, for example, then from day one you are going to be given advice and information about several things, accumulating to around 4-5 topics. So there is so much information and advice to take (especially from the Netherlands) that the days of care do not even make up for how heavy this moment really is and the need to educate is confirmed.

So what is done in other cultures around the world during this time, then you ask? I will speak about my tribe the Mijikenda People, from my first-hand experience and also the wisdom given to me by my female lineage being my maternal aunties, my mother and my grandmother who practised as a traditional midwife within her community for many years.

Within the Mijikenda people, milestones are celebrated from the birth of the baby to the death, concluded with a 40-day celebration or wake, where everyone returns to pray with the family, give blessings and honour their loved one. Because it is a phase we go through that bears a profound impact on our development and growth, every phase in my native country, Kenya, is marked with a celebration.

When a young girl reaches puberty and starts her menstruation cycle, there is a celebration. When the potential husband (serious boyfriend) is introduced to the family, there is a celebration for a wedding and the news of a pregnancy.

The postpartum period is one that is a big event because it concludes the laying-in period for both mother and child. This is the reason Africans, as a people, put a lot of emphasis on this phase: because SHE needs to be protected.

Traditionally, we say life begins with the woman. As the one person who bears life and ensures the continuity of the legacy, she is protected because of the position she holds within a community.

> *Traditionally, only the concerned team was told about the news of a baby coming - Naomie Karemi KAINGU*

Ancestrally, there is a way we have always done things according to the ways of our people. Kenya is a country with 43 different tribes. Each tribe has its ways of doing things, celebrations, and rituals. In this book, I will speak about the tribe I know more about and that is my mother's tribe, the Mijikenda people. The Mijikenda tribe is big with subcategories, too. There are 9 categories, each tribe with its own accent and language too, but from the same Bantu origin meaning many of the words, we can understand each other. These all identify as Mijikenda people. The list comprises the following;

1. Mrabai
2. Mjibana
3. Mchonyi
4. Mkambe
5. Mribe
6. Mdigo
7. Mduruma
8. Mgiriama
9. Mkauma

So the Mijikenda people are tribal people, and their gatherings are not only big but very family-oriented and colorful, too. They are of Bantu origin; the people found in the Coastal part of Kenya, Mombasa, mainly occupying the shores of the Indian Ocean.

They love the warm weather, and fish is their staple food. Isolation and individuality are not something we are comfortable with because we live in communities. We are used to big families living and growing in togetherness. Starting when our daughters marry, we become and identify as one family. You married into the family, and therefore, your well-being was everyone else's responsibility in that village or tribe. From the moment you are trying to conceive, there are already rituals that are performed regarding fertility and preparing the womb to receive and nurture life.

As a tribe, the Mijikenda people have preserved many of their rituals and ways, just like the Maasai who have refused to let go of their hunting for food, basic survival skills that are taught from the moment they are born and wearing 'westernized clothes' as many call them. They still wear their robes, tied differently according to ranking and sex, but their ways are very authentic all throughout the world.

Amongst the Mijikenda people, news of a baby coming brings a whole celebration mood. They believe in returning ancestors, and therefore rituals are prepared before the baby is born even. There are some herbal mixes that a 'king' (midwife) would make for the expectant woman to take throughout the pregnancy for vitality, and also, the herbs have different goodness that one needs to grow and nurture during a pregnancy.

When she is 8 months pregnant, it is expected that she will go back 'home'. Wherever that may be. It may be back to her own parents or the parents-in-law, where she would be cared for during the lying-in period. The expectant parent would normally go back home or where the support system is stronger. I mentioned rituals that are held in preparation.

Each tribe would usually do things according to the ways of their people. I will share briefly about the Mijikenda people, the people from the Coastal part of Kenya who have preserved many of their traditions through generations. Ceremonies are the ways of communicating, gathering together, and concluding RITES within communities.

Because of this also, as a people, we do not announce news of a baby coming. There is an understanding traditionally of why the ancestor coming had to be protected throughout the journey, because it is a journey they travel before they are welcomed back into the family. You will find many in Africa still cover up pregnancy and the news is only shared mostly with '*those concerned.*

How was she supported? It did not mean that she never had a support system should the tides of pregnancy change. It means that the concerned team is there to support them through the entire journey of pregnancy regardless of how it concluded. So in a homestead, care and protectiveness were aimed at the expectant person for several reasons. Africans as a people keep family names and believe that every new life that joins the clan, tribe, or boma (homestead) is a returning ancestor, and therefore their arrival and existence are of great importance in how the legacy expands and grows.

Another reason we are not in favor of baby showers either is that the journey has not concluded and, therefore, 'putting one's eggs in one basket was not encouraged. Amongst the Mijikenda people, they say 'you are mocking God' because the journey is not complete yet to be celebrated. Of course, everyone will do what they want with their pregnancies but understand the ancestral meaning of why it was done this way.

Close family members traveled from far, and many stayed within the homestead until after the 40th-day celebration had been concluded so that by the time all the extra help and support had gone and left you, you could pick up from where you left off and continue to prosper as a family unit. There is also another reason traditionally why only the immediate families could come and see the baby and that is the belief that babies are pure souls.

Anything and everything that evil attracts to everything pure: **babies are pure**. So protection comes for both mother and child because, as a community, protecting what belongs to that legacy was a communal duty. For the lineage to prosper and multiply, we start by looking after the female lineage, because life begins and ends with them.

A celebration of families and friends gathered around after the lying-in period, which was 40 days. Now, depending on your marital status, the newborn mothers got an extra 10 days to prepare them to go back to their marital home not only as mothers, but also as wives. You would have had an extra 'top up' Kamasutra class that included a cooking session, Kamasutra itself, personal hygiene, and more advice or information were explained too.

In Africa, we believe that there are certain parts of animals that men are not fed. Say, for example, a chicken. We do not feed the head of the chicken, so in these classes, you would be taught how and what you can serve your spouse and what not to do, how to look after yourself hygienically, mentally, and physically. Kenya is a country with 43 tribes. Every tribe speaks its own language and has its own rituals and ceremonies. Celebrations are almost similar as in we celebrate dowries, birth, wedding, and death similarly, but the language and the celebrations are held differently.

I will focus mainly on the Mijikenda people who are of Bantu origin and live on the shores of the Indian Ocean in Mombasa, which is the coastal part of Kenya. The Mijikenda people are very cultural and have a particular way of conducting ceremonies.

So because we are on the shores of the ocean, fish is our main meal, as the local fishermen would either know which homes would buy directly from them or they would lay their finds, and people would buy directly from the shores. From the moment the baby is fed, the newborn mother would be fed lean meat, mainly fish and chicken. Every homestead in Kenya rears chicken, so this is very easy to find. It has to be something that her body can digest and still fill her up in aid of milk production.

Milk is also very easy to find because we have farms near many homes and fresh milk is the best. Usually, it would be used in the Chai that would be in a thermos next to her bed or in Millet porridge, which is highly nutritious for lactation, weaning, sick, and the elderly. Another porridge that we add milk to is plain maize-meal porridge. This one is usually served with butter added while it is still warm to add some good fats to a lactating mother

> *The head of the family is the man, but the neck within that homestead is the woman. The head cannot stand by itself, it needs the neck.–African proverb. This is the main reason, culturally, the focus has been on the mother (she/her)*

Birth is a sacred ceremony, and the space within it is protected in a community. When it is time for the baby to be born, the neighboring villages stayed put. Everyone within the homestead is aware of their duties and what they need to be doing to make sure that the process is as stress-free as possible. I was the grandchild who was sent to boil water or get the razor, making sure it was sealed and not broken to cut the cord when the time came.

Traditionally, only a **'concerned'** group was informed of the pregnancy news. A concerned team? Who is the concerned team? You ask. This is the group of people who would stand with you through it all, regardless of how the journey ends. There already was an understanding that birth is an event and therefore anything could happen. Having the '***concerned team*** enabled you to go through it all knowing your support system was there with you throughout. When and if there was a loss, one was supported as needed by this team of people. You got intimate support from people who understood the RITES and traditions and were also old enough to hold space without making you feel some kind of way.

As you journey through pregnancy, birth, and postpartum, be mindful of the energy you welcome in your space. A womb being blessed is not a given. Not everyone who prays to the same God you prayed to was granted a pregnancy. Therefore, news of such a blessing was kept low until it was time to reveal the blessing and only with the concerned group of people. Be mindful of who you share news of pregnancy because even ancestrally there was an understanding that even amongst us there are folk we laugh with every day going through infertility who have not shared their anguish with us all. People are going through reproductive problems that they are not sharing with us, so your news may not be 'good' news for everyone, and that is not the energy you need either

Another reason we need to know who we invite in our midst is that regardless of how the birth developed and came to conclude, you need people who will see your need for support and will offer it without a hunchback. A support network that understands that you do not just support when it's a happy ending, but also what being supporting means. You need the support of people who see you in the pit of emotions, but do not keep you there with pity because it is very easy to remain on the 'oh my word, oh poor you' wagon, offering no solution.

You need the support of those who would offer you their hand and say, " Hold on to this hand, I am going to help you out and when you are on this other side, we can find a solution as we support you through it. In the current times, many don't know how to support others. Be mindful of who you ask for support and what kind of support you need from them. For some, even the people we have done life with and guaranteed they would be around, their support is a debt that will be slapped back to your face.

Ancestrally, this is the reason outside influence and energy were guarded. The entire community had a duty to ensure that nobody that does not belong within wandered around because of various reasons I will explain as you continue reading. The protection of the lineage was very important for the lineage (family line) because Africans, as a people, keep family names.

The moment the expectant person arrives back home to her homestead, be it the parents-in-laws or her own parents, to prepare for the birth of the baby, herbs that need to be gathered would usually be gathered, barks that need to be boiled to make tinctures would be done in readiness, and her 'manyatta' (mud hut with a sisal roof or grass) would be ready as her birthing shrine. The immediate moments after the birth of a baby are a time for 'nothingness' where the birthing person is still lingering spiritually and hasn't landed yet.

There is a lot of adjusting that is demanded at this moment, and the openness of the spiritual space at this moment is very sacred. The importance of this moment and its sacredness is something that many young people grow up learning because you see that within the community. Research has confirmed something that ancestrally has always been done. A pregnant brain is a real thing.

When she returned to prepare for the birth, she was paired with another lady of age who she could call for help if needed. That second person would become their second brain as their body worked extra hard in preparation, and forgetfulness became part of the pregnancy. Her paired companion became her second brain, so that whatever was shared or spoken regarding the birth did not pass her.

You do not have to justify or fight for everyone around you to understand your need to recuperate or recover after childbirth. Everybody understood the need for nothing to happen whilst you recovered, learned your baby's cues, adjusted, and connected as a family without distraction.

Close family members traveled from far, and many stayed within the homestead until after the 40th-day celebration had been concluded so that by the time all the extra help and support had gone and left, they could pick up and continued to prosper as a family unit. There was also another reason traditionally why only immediate families could come and see the baby in the immediate postpartum, and that is the belief that *babies are pure souls.* Ancestrally, it is said that anything that is pure attracts everything that is evil.

Babies are pure, hence the protection over them because they cannot do that for themselves.

So, protection is for both mother and child because, as a community, protecting what belongs to that legacy was a communal duty. For the lineage to prosper and multiply, we start by looking after the female lineage, because life begins and ends with them. The protectiveness stems from the belief that the man is the head of the family. His wife/partner/other half is the neck that the head needs. The neck has to be protected for the neck to stand, and without it, the head cannot stand. It is just as important as the head of a clan or tribe.

Women are not only respected, but they are also part of the deciding committee. Therefore, having their approval passed you within a tribe.

Three

FIRST THEY WERE UNVEILED

Some tasks were only done once and others were throughout the postpartum lying-in, like body scrubs and massages offered daily. The Mkunga or your maternal mother would suggest steaming when the bleeding stops to help cleanse and close the cycle. Naturally, a newborn mother (she/her) could come back to herself from her spiritual journey.

It is believed that she went to, leaving her body to fetch her baby and bring them back; earth-side. Traditionally, the roar of the birthing mother meant she was instinctively connecting with her mammal self so that she could go deep within herself to seek strength. Then she would return more robust than before she left, ready to birth her baby fearlessly, intuitively, and in her power.

When she showed signs of being **present**, the older person within the Manyatta whispered her name in the ear to call her back in the now.

What does the unveiling mean? Let me start by explaining something my grandmother made me understand even after having my third child. She described an uncertain feeling. I could not explain it in words. Many people cannot identify it. The transition occurs between the **RITES** of passages, from the moment you start your first period to the moment you test positive for a pregnancy and then the last part where you give birth and become a parent. A considerable change happens when a young lady transitions from matrescence (the physical, emotional, hormonal, and social growth for young girls) into motherhood or parenting.

During this transition phase, the young woman crosses from one norm to another.

> We were never intended to go through the **RITES** of passage alone.

The unveiling helps the birthing person understand it may seem easy when they are still pregnant, but it is not. Nobody is born a mother or a parent, and it is something that we learn and see around us growing up. We were our elders' mirrors, and we remember we are our next generation's mirrors, too. What we normalize and allow them to see is the only truth they will know. It is hard work but rewarding, and all the wisdom amongst the expectant parents becomes of good use.

Well, when we think of everything else' 'consent' or everything introduced to the big world, there is a ceremony of cutting the ribbon. There is usually a grand opening, and then the item is available to be bought and used. Why aren't women unveiled? What does it mean to be **unveiled**? The unveiling is more like consent in the modern world. In Swahili, we say '*Mficha uchi hazai*, meaning those who hide their nakedness cannot birth nor be served.

The unveiling is part of why there were gatherings to go through the importance of allowing others to care for you and be of service to you and your baby in your most vulnerable and open mode of being.

The older women would share stories about their own experiences and what support looked like for them. The shared stories helped you appreciate and understand that this RITE of passage is one that many of you have gone through as well. Stories were told by the elders to the pregnant women within the clan to instill confidence and resilience as they approached the phase of being parents.

Stories meant to help you see that a whole village of wisdom was around you because many who came in readiness for the birth of your baby stayed until after your 40 days celebration concluded, so you were guaranteed to have community support through the RITE of passage that is childbirth.

The unveiling was a ceremony attended by women only because women supported and stood for each other through the RITES of childbirth and the immediate postpartum. Your mother or mother-in-law would delegate tasks, and your focus remained on being rested.

TOUCH

The benefit of touch is it brings a sense of care and wellness to newborn mothers. In my native country Kenya, newborn mothers (they/she) are wrapped and then massaged with warm towels and clothes. Naturally, heat helps with healing and also helps with blood flow in areas that are injured or stagnant because of shock. A person who has given birth aches and their body is also shocked. The organs must shift back to their respective positions, where they pave the way for the baby to emerge.

She would lie on a bed made with sisal threads; underneath it would be pots of herbs to help steam her from the bottom up.

Massages bring warmth to the body, which helps with recovery. They are being massaged, seated upright on a hard wooden stool which allows the perineum to heal.

On the three stones where fire has been burning from the morning, there would be a clay pot that is heated, wrapped with a cloth, and then put on the lower part of the stomach to bring heat right through to the back of the body. After the massage, a warm towel is used to rub her down, another heated pair of khanga is used to wrap her up, and then the last part is the **Dera** covers her up completely

SOUND/VOICE

In the immediate postpartum period, tribes and female lineage would sing family or clan songs known for uplifting and encouragement. As small children, we grew up hearing these songs sung around us for generations. Outside the Manyatta, there would be drum and horning, and the male elders were already with Palm Wine. Fires would burn around the 'boma' or homestead to invite ancestors who have died before us and warm up the children gathering around it to listen to the elders' stories every evening after everyone has eaten. So birth is celebrated from day one like this.

The baby is spoken to as if they understood from the first moment. The grandmother who would have been in the birthing hut or Manyatta would talk to the child's ear like they were passing a message because the baby is still wandering, finding their environment.

The wandering is said to signify that a baby is looking for its lineage, and the messages shared with the baby allow them to arrive home. Then the maternal grandmother or an elder from the Manyatta would announce the birth to the community, leaving the Manyatta from the right-hand side if the baby was a boy and from the left if the baby was female.

BREASTFEEDING

The wise women within the tribe taught the art of breastfeeding in the first moments of nesting. As young girls, women saw others around them breastfeed, saw the support given to breastfeeding mothers too, and understood why breastfeeding was important. Ancestrally breastfeeding was given until the baby stopped by themselves. My mother breastfed our last born until he was four years old. In the current times, research tells us that a mother's milk contains a lot of nutrients and vital vitamins for the growing baby. Ancestrally, it was the only food fed to babies, understanding that mother's milk was also crucial for a growing baby without scientific reasons.

Though natural, nursing a baby is an art that a newly birthed mother has to learn. It is not something you know simply by being born female. Your baby's cues would help you know when they have had enough and when to feed them again. The guidance was done from day one until the young parents-to-be understood the art and importance of breastfeeding, and then support was offered as and when needed. Breastfeeding was adored and encouraged by others. Previously, if women went back to work in the fields, wet nursing was encouraged only then babies who fed from the same breast could never marry when they grew up.

Holding positions were explained to you, how to care for your breasts to avoid infections between mother and child, and how to massage the breasts when they eventually filled with milk were shown. Africans, as a people, are taught or learned through stories shared during age-appropriate gatherings. The older generation passed down information that would equip the young generation. It was shown by examples and narrated as a story.

The staple food for a breastfeeding parent was Maize meal porridge or porridge made with a mix of grains or Millet and milk known for being lactogenic (stimulates and increases prolactin levels). The focus would also be on staple roots like cassava, cooked in coconut cream and served with fried fish like Red snapper.

FOOD/DIET

The food one eats after birth is vital, as some foods may cause constipation and swelling of certain parts, like the perineum and the legs. The system goes dormant, almost in shock, and it all has to restart functioning. Aside from being massaged, the newborn mother was fed many vegetables like spinach, okra, and lentils (Mung Beans) to help against constipation. The kitchen team would cook many grains like mung beans or lentils in coconut cream, which is lactogenically known ancestrally.

In Mombasa, the staple food is fish; therefore, the postpartum person's meals would comprise a lot of fish. One main fish dish is the soup of Octopus, which is said to help maintain the libido of both genders after childbirth. Fish is also lean to digest. Ugali (maize meal cake, if you like) is also our staple food. Usually cooked hard, it is in the early weeks after birth cooked soft and palatable. Lots of green vegetables would be prepared and served to the newly birthed mother to help combat constipation and help them flush their kidneys.

The postpartum person would have prepared spinach, Moringa, and beans with gas removed. In Kenya, when we cook beans, they would be washed before the cooking started, and then the first water whilst they are still cooking would be disposed of several times.

The water that is dark is poured out at least 3 times before the beans are completely cooked.

Aside from water served either warm or at room temperature, coconut water, also known for flushing the kidneys while nourishing them, was served to her. The coconut would be picked young, not mature, because the younger the coconut, the better the flavor of the meat inside and the more water inside it. Today, coconut water helps energize a birthing person because it re-hydrates, has enough calories, and contains suitable electrolytes.

The postpartum clan looking after her would scoop the coconut meat from the coconut for her to eat. Coconuts are chosen 'young' so that the inside remains slippery, which helps with constipation and is filling.

Baked bananas would be cooked with thick coconut cream to boost breastfeeding and sweet combat cravings. For sweet cravings, the team in the kitchen would also cook ripe bananas. They would be drizzled with warming spices like Cardamom and Cinnamon to warm her up, always served with a spicy cup of Chai. Roasted nuts would also be in plenty, like cashews roasted in the ground, and the fruit served in pieces for her to eat fresh.

Four

THEN THEY WERE WELCOMED AND HONOURED

The welcoming was the following step that had to happen before the closing and the celebration. With the welcome, immediate female lineage came to congratulate you in your postpartum bed, show support, and offer help where needed ahead of the final celebrations. The welcoming happened in the second part of the process because it takes a while to leave the 'hello' zone to becoming, and you must be supported through the transition so that it is not too overwhelming, which can be like it and quickly too.

The welcoming ensured that you had 'landed' and were healthy, responding to your baby's needs and that mentally you were stable, too. In this mode, you can receive information and engage by asking questions. You were honored amongst your tribe for surviving the process and referred to with your new title **mama x**

HOW TO SIT - THE POSTPARTUM PREPARATION

Many do not know the wisdom of how a postpartum person is to sit. They are never spoken about unless you meet someone with an ancestral background and knowledge. Did you know that how you sit after childbirth can also alter your sex life and well-being afterward? In the current times, the focus is on the pelvic floor. Women are coached beforehand on exercising after childbirth to help the pelvic floor muscles not only for their sexual lives after birth but because the pelvic floor must be trained and toned; otherwise, you hear of women who leak urine when they laugh or cough and others who leak because the muscles were too damaged to be repaired or too injured to train.

Ancestrally, wise women taught pregnant women the importance of caring for their perineum before childbirth. Once your bleeding decreased, steaming was encouraged to help emit what could not leave your body naturally. Okra is a vegetable served the last week of the due date to help change the vaginal discharge so that the surrounding area becomes wet and slippery. When a woman is ready to give birth, one herb used to help make the perineum firm but flaccid is one we call *'mkone'* from the leaves of a coconut tree. It is pounded in a certain way and used to rinse the perineum after every toilet visit until after birth.

In the postpartum period, where you spend 100 percent of your time in bed, you are shown how to sit. A person who has birthed life should not sit with their legs wide open, even under the bedsheets when you connect the fact that once you have given birth, everything remains open from the womb where the placenta detached; therefore, the whole womb is empty and prone to infections, etc. When the air gets inside the womb in the first weeks after childbirth, it may come out eventually, but wise women would educate on the importance of not allowing air to get inside from the word go. Many women complain about this air or wind later on that they feel like they are farting through the day from their vaginas.

This wind can, for some women, be a permanent problem where it affects their sex life in that they fart from their vaginas.

BATH/SHOWER

Ancestrally newborn mothers could not drench in water from head to toe. They were encouraged to keep and maintain their body temperatures and stay dry. Washing or bathing, the newly birthed mother was done after the 40th day of the postpartum period. Every aspect of the woman's body remains physically and spiritually open after birth. Even on a continent as hot as Africa, newly birthed mothers could not wash or shower.

Knowing that after childbirth your uterus remains open and the wound where your placenta had nourished and took care of your baby from within detaches, you can imagine you will need a little more time to heal from within. The wound from within demands that you slow down and take your rest with every opportunity. Because of this, you are prone to catching infections and colds. The **mkunga** would prepare warm water mixed with salt, which you would be used for rinsing after using the bathroom. The mix is used to relieve swelling, cuts, or trauma in the perineum and was only used to rinse yourself after going to the toilet.

A little is also used on the head, mixed with coconut oil, to rub you down after a body massage and scrubs. Otherwise, you remain dry, keeping your body temperature, and the aura helps comfort a newborn baby until your official wash, where an older aunt would wash you down with herbs before your post-laying in celebration. Bathing the baby was also delayed because the body has natural fats, and washing and then rubbing the skin was discouraged until after the umbilical cord had detached.

A ceremony was performed to bury the dried navel string and pray for the fertility lineage. How the navel cord falls is very important for both boys and girls. It should never fall in the middle of the body but on the sides. The navel string/cord falling in the middle of the body meant that fertility lineage could be affected culturally.

Five

FINALLY THEY WERE CLOSED AND CELEBRATED

Ancestrally, the health and recovery of the birthing mother were vital within a tribe or community. The news or thought of her not surviving the phase of childbirth and then the postpartum period was devastating to the community. Her recovery and well-being meant that the legacy and lineage continued to be extended. Life begins with birth, so her health and recovery were a communal investment.

The closing is done throughout the postpartum period in bits depending on the birth event and where the birthing person is mentally. Sometimes it is conducted over a more extended period, but we will focus on this phase after childbirth. From the moment the baby was born, the mother would be massaged and rubbed down using clay and a cleansing stone we call *'liwa'* used for weddings to cleanse and purify the skin. Liwa is like a turmeric root, which is also orange and would be rubbed repeatedly on a slab with some water to create a paste that is then used directly on the skin.

She remained in her birthing hut until she was ready to move back into the family home, usually around the 20th day when she was more stable and bleeding less. In the mud hut, she was resting on a bed made of sisal, where a pot of boiling herbs steamed her through the bed's gaps and helped ease body aches instead of laying on a soft mattress.

Whenever she was being rubbed down with the herbs and cleansing pastes, she would sit on a wooden stool, a hard surface, to help put pressure on her perineum and also to help strengthen her pelvic floor. Her belly and hips would be massaged gently and then wrapped daily to help her weak and unstable joints recover to their rightful place. The instability of joints is a complaint that many women and birthing people complain about childbirth, the instability of their pelvis and joints. Ancestrally, it was understood that the womb carrying life could expand and that it could be molded back to help with recovery.

Typically, in an African setting where someone has given birth, there is a pot on three stones over a fire that burns the whole time. It is filled with new firewood and the pots over the fire to cook day and night. Water is used for various uses, from making soups and teas mixed with salt and other herbs to rinsing yourself after using the toilet, rubbing her body down, rinsing her nipples before feeding the baby and after, and for many other uses. The fire burns throughout because it is understood that babies are born cold. Also, fire burning is used to keep the Manyatta (African sisal and clay birthing hut) warm because the birthing person is open and prone to catching colds.

Ancestrally, there was an understanding that a pregnant woman's bones expanded to pave the way for the baby's growth and helped to birth the baby. Binding her helped mold her back into a stable structure. They were then 'ready for the next pregnancies, as my grandmother would say. She was bound every day for 40 days and sometimes even longer, while some continued binding a year or two into their parenting journey.

Within the Manyatta, her postpartum team used warm water to massage her hair daily. Massaging her hair helps to avoid postpartum hair loss. Hair follicles are massaged with coconut oil mixed with warm water every day, and then her hair is braided or plated down with enough oil smeared in a protective style away from her face or breasts. Her mother or Mkunga would also use water mixed with coconut oil. Water mixed with coconut oil penetrates the skin better than on its own. Putting hair in protective styles in the postpartum period is also deemed to help eliminate hair loss. Hair massages are given after good deep towel steam, where the hair follicles are pampered and oiled.

The newly birthed person would not pour water over her body for 40 days. The only contact they had with water was from the massages received because they are believed to be very open after birth and in the fragile postpartum weeks. Therefore, to protect them from catching a cold, they stayed dry and only rinsed the parts that needed to be flushed, like her perineum, where she would be taught the frequency of changing the pad and what to look out for her breasts to wade of making the baby sick.

THE CEREMONY

The 40-day celebration is the excellent part of things, and a lot of work goes into ensuring it is successful. In Mombasa, festivals are colorful and enormous. They mostly last a few to seven days in total. Every day there is a different theme leading to the concluding day. Every day, folk gather to unite, eat, drink and wait for the reveal day when they will officially meet the new mother and her baby. There is a lot of drumming, songs, cheers, and prayers. Right through the last pregnancy stages, plans are made as standby for what ceremony would befit the baby that would be born. Depending on who they are named after and if that person is still alive, the grandness is decided upon that information. If it is a baby girl named after their grandmother, you can expect something grand, just like if they were a baby boy named after their grandfather and what number of grandchildren they are too. As the ceremony approached, there were big plans for the coming day.

Inside the separate household that houses the new mother and her baby, she receives the same treatments she has received throughout the laying-in period leading to the day of her revelation. She is massaged, her skin rubbed with salts and homemade pastes, her hair moisturized, steamed, and then she is closed with khanga. The closing ceremony entails the baby's father being present because there are prayers and specific words that the elders of the family unit share. The partner is then invited to boast and bless his partner for a job well done. He would have gathered gifts for her, sometimes as jewelry or a herd like a male and female sheep or cow, that would represent his adoration for her.

After the laying-in days are finished, the celebration occurs. The whole community, near and far, comes to you to introduce the baby and congratulate the new parents and grandparents. The celebration is one aspect of the birth that is discussed months ahead of the birth. Materials; such as herbs, tinctures, livestock, and clothes like African prints, are gathered and chosen for the ceremony so that visitors would also know who is family and friends are and who from the gathering is a guest.

The 40-day celebration is one that is planned for ahead of time like a wedding, where attention to detail is key, from the songs that will be played, the speeches and who will speak, the instruments or gifts that the immediate family will gather depending on the gender of the baby, palm wine had to be ordered from the best sellers ahead of time so that they prepared the best. Fruits and roots are gathered ahead of time, and community posts are allocated.

Everyone within the clan will know beforehand their position or task on this day. Planning for this day begins much earlier into the pregnancy because prints, especially certain prints, you can only buy at certain times of the year.

The prints are chosen intentionally to symbolize something, especially the khanga we (Eastern Africans) use throughout our adult lives. The print on the khanga can be printed with a chosen message or words.

People availed themselves to attend this special day of initiation. Prayers are sent to the newborn family, especially the baby; everyone who comes is allowed to carry the baby. Finally, the elders and the parents would introduce the baby to the extended family on this day. They would meet their lineage and be welcomed officially into the community. That would be the day the new parents would be welcomed back into the community, and the birthing person or Mother (She/her) she would be brought out like a bride. That would be the day that almost everyone welcomed would hold the baby and offer their prayer and well-wishes as they grew up.

The newborn mother would be celebrated as a fellow mother amongst her peers and the community. The new mother would sit next to her female peer, who is also married during the blessings part; then she would be joined by her partner and children, if any. Her dress is chosen to be unique amongst the rest of the attendees so that she stands out. African people are very proud of their prints. Therefore, preparations leading to this day are held with utmost importance because everything has to be perfect on this day.

The elders choose words that are usually printed at the bottom of **Khanga**, depending on the gender of the baby, who they would be named after, and their namesake rank within the community.

The words are chosen to mean something significant or to iterate something that the baby's namesake would have done, like being a leader or having held a specific ranking within the tribe. Sometimes the words are also picked as blessings under the child's name. When the celebration starts, the new parents would be introduced back to the community with their new titles.

We usually call parents according to their children's names. So, for example, if your firstborn child is Sandra, then you would be known as **'mama Sandra** and **baba Sandra.**

After this celebration, the couple can mate and continue their marital duties. There will be the talk of when the kitchen party would be held, a celebration that is women only where the new mother (She/Her) is taught again how to prepare certain meals in the kitchen, how to look after her home, her husband now as a mother and also as a wife.

Traditionally, certain parts of a chicken, for example, are not fed to the man of the house. So a kitchen party is like a resit class, and then she is also gifted her waistbands, with beads that are chosen symbolically for the family's prosperity. The colors are intentionally selected for her, and the man has a separate gathering to teach him how to use the beads, especially those intended for his use as a husband within their private chambers.

Six

SUPPORT STARTS FROM WITHIN

... the home before it is outsourced - Naomie Karemi KAINGU

This part here surprises many: Postpartum support does not need to cost an arm and a leg to conclude. You can have a wholesome postpartum period simply by planning and having open discussions with those you love and respect beforehand.

Use the collective of friends and neighbors willing to be of support to you in your immediate postpartum period and be willing to receive. Be open to being supported, held, and carried in your most vulnerable moment because people are willing, but most times, newborn parents reject support with the notion that all is under control. Whilst that may be the case, the postpartum period brings with it many hurdles and surprises and you are better off having a backup of people you can count on to be available when you need them. It is one of the most unpredictable moments in your life, simply as birth.

You cannot plan beforehand that the baby will keep a good weight and be able to control their body temperature, for example.

Or that your baby will not get jaundice, which is common in the first week, and sometimes the baby needs to be admitted to the hospital for treatment. Having a baby is not just hard work, it is mentally, emotionally, and physically exhausting.

Discuss beforehand and find out directly the support that is expected of you so that it is not a surprise when you are in the neck of things. In the postpartum period, the support network starts from within the home, and within the community (family, friends, acquaintances, neighbors, etc) before you seek outside. Understandably, it is not a given to have folk around who will drop everything at your mercy, then it becomes teamwork and effort between you both.

> *Understand that REST is important, she is not being lazy when you see her lying down–Naomie Karemi KAINGU*

Even for you as a partner, realize that, just because they said she could go home from the hospital, does not mean she has *'landed'*. Many times, there are doors that are not yet closed. The mental load of a birthing person remains full for a long time. She may have heard things, made to feel a certain way, or told words that cut deep, words that hurt so much, that she chose not to speak about, swept them under the carpet, and never spoke about them because she dealt with that in this way.

Those are the things we automatically never question because the person carrying that load is the same person everybody else relies on to be available and almost immediately, to feed her baby, to receive information, that nobody stops to think maybe, just maybe, her own load is too heavy for her to carry.

Just because she is looking good (because come on, some people are born artists and they can slap that make-up so good you would never guess they have issues) does not mean that she IS feeling good. Remember that those living within the home are the ones who see the level of support needed before they source for outside help. Regardless of how the birth developed, her strength comes from being held and supported through her recovery period. There is a reason ancestrally this was done, and it is the invisible physical and mental workload that comes with being 'mama'.

Her birth could have been the worst for all the onlookers, but as long as she is held through so she can piece everything together and process it, she will conquer it to a certain degree. Having the right support can change how the future unfolds for you as a family, too. With the right support, even the hardest future is one that you know you will travel to alone. There is something to be said about people who walk to accompany you through this life. She will not find her ground and 'land' calmly if those around her 24/7 are not supportive.

She will fail in breastfeeding, for example, unless those around her recognize that breastfeeding, though natural, is hard work and their support is vital for her to establish, learn, and succeed in the breastfeeding journey. If only she has to remember everything else, including her own well-being, then some things she will not achieve because one cannot create 6 versions of themselves without crumbling. So those who are within and around her need to know that outside support will only be available for 8 hours at the most and after that, she will be left with her immediate circle.

Protect each other - as a birth partner, your support in postpartum is needed even more. So, protect her space like you did the birthing room. She needs to know you are her support system both mentally, and emotionally and when the tough gets going, she can come to you for refuge. When there is the absence of the 'village' and the willingness of others, you are her greatest support.

When she is fragile, open, emotional, and struggling, see what you can do to support her settlement. Don't forget yourself in taking care of your own needs, and checking in with each other through parenting is vital. You are a team and inevitably sometimes you will not agree, but both your first priorities are with each other. Allow the friends who could support you too, so that you can support each other properly. Just like at birth, if unsure, always ask until it makes sense for you.

Be true to both of you - if you know that your immediate family will not support her the way she needs to be supported. Men see things differently, especially where their own mothers are concerned. Women have a tendency to shame others naturally, and In this moment and time, your main priority is your partner/girlfriend/wife.

Think of the 9 months when she nurtured, carried, and then birthed your baby when you could only connect with the baby in vitro, and quite different from how she did. Once the baby is born, your priority should be to establish and connect with your family

Importance of Education/knowledge - Education beforehand is important so that she can be sure that the partners will not utter words that will not be encouraging to her recovery. If you see her resting is because she needs to rest, especially those first few weeks, so that she can continue functioning when all the extra hands have left and life has to continue.

Breastfeeding takes a lot of energy out of you and just because the baby is thriving does not mean she is not worn out. And sometimes it will not be something that she will enjoy doing because it is not fun all the time with breastfeeding.

Partners need to be brought in, in the world of pregnancy, birth, Postpartum, and bereavement too, to understand that as fathers and as partners, they ARE the primary gatekeepers.

And that whilst in that position, they are, in fact, in the gateways of both life and death. Her strength will not come from being supported. She would thaw and deflate and the spite that evaporates in this phase is one that is hard to resolve, even with therapy. So be aware that you are in this together as a team.

She needs you to do more than just tidy up because, mostly, her role as a mother is very invisible and will remain so always.

Be involved - in all the planning because this is a journey for you both and what may have worked in your friend 'Charley's house' may not work in yours. Being involved in the planning enables you to understand also the invisible load that she has to prepare for as you get ready to welcome a new baby. Being involved means you will know what to do should 'life' happen, or she ends up staying in the hospital for whatever reason. Especially when there are other children.

Know their agendas, their activities, when what happens, and what to pack, and ask if it is not clear.

Stories and other people's experiences are to enlighten certain parts of some things that may well be a reality to others, but please know that someone else's story is not your reality. By being involved in the planning, you are inevitably allowing yourself to be useful should you need to. Imagine something happens, and she ends up staying in the hospital for a considerable amount of time. You, being at home, need to know what happens when she is doing it all, where everything is in case you get asked to bring something when something happens, like the other children's activities and so on.

Plan - Having a plan throughout your pregnancy, the birth and even a postpartum plan clears things out ahead of time. This way you will know what your role is in all the phases, what is expected of you, and also how to be supportive. When you make a plan beforehand things are spoken about ahead of time, if you can not support them fully because by x time you would be gone back to work then you can plan for her to be supported by someone else, but then it is agreed upon by both parties and the extra help appointed ahead of time.

> *Planning for your postpartum is better than winging it. Naomie Karemi KAINGU.*

If you decide to outsource help, be mindful that they are in line with your family's needs and virtues. For example, if you do not eat meat, then you want someone who knows not to cook it in your home. Explain what is important for your family and the support you need and hope to receive ahead of time.

It will not cook itself - Now I see this a lot with my brothers sometimes when I visit postpartum homes. Her needing support does not mean you going up to the supermarket, stocking up the fridge, and then chilling because that food will not cook itself. If cooking is a task for you, know a restaurant near you that delivers wholesome meals.

These days Hello fresh can really save the day because they send a complete package of what makes up a meal and they are usually fast recipes. If your own immediate family is around, plan an evening where they can come and batch-cook food that you can freeze up so that it is ready to warm up and serve. If you have a postpartum doula, speak about the number of hours they can come and see if you can set up a meal train amongst your friends and family so that people can support you in this way until you find your own strength.

The postpartum period can be many things, but the truth of the matter is; that it is all about reintroducing yourself to yourself. Slowly finding your own pace, your own ground, your own balance as a family. Integrating into a rhythm with each other and especially when there are other children, they all need to find their own places within the family unit and therefore a lot of calm, understanding, and patience is paramount.

Cut the cliches - Don't keep hitting her with lines like ' babe you are so good at this, she will chew you up! Nobody taught her how to parent and you need to pull your own socks and stand to be seen. Parenting is a journey. Together, you will conquer it. It takes a lot of understanding that there is no good cop-bad cop, but that you are a team.

Compliment her not because you want to run away from the duties, but because she really deserves the compliments. There are many things you can do to support and ease the transition that you cannot do naturally, like breastfeeding the baby.

1. Lay a tray and refill it with things that don't spoil throughout the day
2. Make sure there is a drink even if just water after she is finished breastfeeding or a thermos of tea
3. Have healthy snacks near her
4. Help feed the baby at night with a bottle so that she can top up and preserve her energy for the night feeds
5. Whilst she is breastfeeding, sterilize the bottles ready for the night feeding (that you will help with)

6. Top up the changing table with diapers, wipes, and 1 set of clothes for when they are needed
7. Take the baby away from her so that she can switch off and rest. Many mothers do not sleep through with their babies near
8. Help burp the baby for example after every feed so that she can drink or feed herself too
9. Be present in providing physical support like belly binding through the postpartum period
10. Compliment her for every milestone she has conquered and continues to

In this way, you not only help her feel she has a little breathing space, that you enabled her to breathe by herself, but you are also learning about your baby, know what comforts them, how to comfort them, soak into the baby mode and really connect with your little person

Body shame or embarrassment is something that many women feel after childbirth. And then.. let her tell you she is ready after the 6 weeks of recovery time. Many men literally count the dates and wait eagerly to go back to their marital duties. Understand that there would be many doubts and she may even be scared because her body image has changed, she would still leak milk, and also most probably not be able to do some positions she used to pre-pregnant. *Remember that your children are an addition to what you two are about. They stem from the two of you. So don't forget yourselves in the mix and tangle of parenting.*

> *Be patient and encourage her also that you embrace her change. Her changed body nurtured and birthed your little one. Honour her please*

Seven

SUPPORT COMES FROM PEOPLE WHO SEE YOUR NEED

… to be supported and are willing to offer it. I love to encourage family members to support and be involved, especially where childbirth and raising legacies are concerned, but for many reasons, it may not be an option for some families. Unfortunately for others, there are toxic family members and then you have to decide what is best for your family situation

> *Support comes from those who see your need for support and are willing to offer it. Naomie Karemi KAINGU*

Sometimes those we hold and love dearly are not the ones who will support us in fragile times for various reasons. You are better off getting help from outside when you doubt if you really will be supported in your most slow and intimate recovery moment. Paid individuals many times will do their work and support you diligently as opposed to a close relative who might have a different out view or expectation from you

Her recovered brain - Towards the end of the pregnancy, many women become very forgetful because there is so much to plan and do, and also the thinking part of the brain kind of takes a back seat, I think. In this mode, she will let anything that does not serve her go because she needs to focus on things that matter. Her energy is demanded to finish the race of nurturing the baby and for many, this is the moment you can get away with so much with them. Be mindful that it is not something that cuts deep through her because it will be the national anthem in your home.

And so, just like pregnancy spikes the hormones, you hear they sense a lot of things and from remarkable distances too, her brain will never forget how she was made to feel in this moment. Many times, with subsequent pregnancies, what did not happen or happened last time is what you will hear. Everything that you were not, and she did not like, would come out when you are preparing for the following birth. This goes to show that their memory is still very much alert and these moments can affect how they continue as parents.

Prioritize yourself first - Meet your baby and connect with your family first before letting others do that. As a birthing person, you give light to your partner he/she returns it to you. You need space to do this without others meddling in between. Remember, the connection is with you three/four within the home first. For 9 months she has done a lot of connecting with the baby in utero. It is your turn to bond with your baby and connect with them in your presence, and that demands time. So make sure you are ok to have the moments you could bond to host and share with others. This is prone to fathers because there is beauty in seeing their mothers with their grandchildren.

Do not forget that your baby needs to build a bond with you first. After the mother comes, you are the father and now that the baby is in your arms; you have all the time and ability to build a connection you couldn't do in utero. When the time comes, and you are ready to outsource help, please use a few of the tips here for your own peace of mind

Be mindful of the energy you welcome around you, regardless of how the birth evolved. There is a thing called 'Toxic positivity'. When someone is too positive and you are not yet ready to hear their 'positive' story yet, it can rub you the wrong way and bring some awkwardness into the space. Some people can not help themselves from sharing, but you can also choose how you would like to receive such kinds of stories. How you receive the information matters because, if you are ready, you can deal with your emotions diligently. If you are not ready, speak with your maternity nurse and ask if they can be around to listen out and correct where needs corrections are needed. Everyone has a story, but for many, letting other people make sense of their own stories does not come naturally.

Validate her feelings - For many women and birthing persons, being touched in front of their loved ones can feel a bit violating and shameful even. Sometimes the midwife would need to check for dilation when they can not find the information right away. If you are present for many, it is not a sight they want to see. Necessary as it may have been, it is still not the same as if you touched them. Understand that she may have a sense of shame about the fact that happened in front of you. If you talk about things openly, it will elevate the awkward feeling afterwards and allow her to normalize that. That part was not in her control and it had to happen

Check what the supporter's understanding of the fourth trimester is - Make sure they understand the needs of a newborn mother and child, whether instinctually or by training she has attended so that you are not bringing stress on top of stress if that is the case. Make sure they know what is needed at this moment and time. Interview them together and if it does not feel right, interview another until you find your match.

Yourself: Don't forget YOU as a father/partner/husband/boyfriend. Don't forget to catch your own breath and fill your own lungs, too. Loving from the overflow applies not only to the mother or the other parent, it applies to you both. Sometimes, throughout the experience of parenting, you will find you need to give each other space. It is very natural that you learn to accept what is at hand and go with the flow a little. Setting expectations and too many of them will have you both flopping in no time. Babies sometimes cry and they cry a lot for no apparent reason. They may have dry diapers, be fed, not sick, and still cry.

Breathe: Take a moment for yourself, even if it's to walk around the block alone and come back in. You will find that changing scenery and being away from each other creates a shift and change in energies that you were not even aware you both needed. Parenting is eternal, and it is a job that comes with many hurdles, trials, and tribulations, too. It is a long journey. Breathe through it. When you stop to breathe, you give yourself time to pause. When you pause, you can regroup and bring in a bit of clarity.

It won't make sense to others: But.. Only you two will understand why you set out what, and why it works for you. Parenting has a way of waking up '*the professors*' amongst us and others even get hurt by having their opinions rejected or called out. Parenting and what you set up within your family unit will ONLY make sense to you.

Sometimes it is better - to hire someone from outside who is not emotionally attached to you to support your family. Unfortunately, there are mothers who do not know how to love or support their own children, flesh and blood. Sometimes your family may feel belittled in this aspect that you sourced help from outside, but it is always better this way. Many times, even those who are 'our own' don't know how to support us. Hiring someone guarantees that you will be supported professionally and referred to if need be. The problem with having only extended family giving support is there is always a feeling of entitlement and ridicule when they are around. Some people simply don't know how to support others

> *They would weaponize the fact that they were around when you needed support at every opportunity possible.*

The postpartum period is a period for the birthing person to recover. If people around her will not help her achieve this, they are better off away so that she can gather herself and recuperate because if nothing changes, birth will. This is not a moment for her to be tip-toeing around people either for fear of 'hurting their feelings. Her hormones will be all over the place, and she may not even be gentle with herself or you, her partner. Adding extending family in the mix is something you need to both agree upon and carefully

This is part of the reason ancestrally why the women went back home until after the postpartum period had ended and they were healed. Maybe not fully, but they had rest and peace for those immediate six weeks after childbirth

Eight

WHEN YOU VISIT...

Be ok with seeing the newly birthed parent or mother lying in bed, that they are not the ones who opened the door for you.

> *Understand that a birthing person NEEDS rest, love, nurturing, and care, NOT gifts.*

Allow her to rest and not be your host the moment you visit. Allow her to be where she is at that you find her without judgment. Normalize hearing that other parents are tired even if you soldiered on in your time. Allow her to experience this moment at her pace, her own way, without you projecting your ideas or experience into hers. Be mindful of the space you enter, because, in the immediate postpartum, they are still in their 'hello cloud' getting to know each other as a couple again, as a family, and as parents. Your comments are not needed at this moment.

Don't turn up with a bagful of gifts wrapped in wrapping paper, empty-handed. Regardless of your family lineage and whether you breastfed yourself if you are her mother, newborn mothers **NEED**

food to make milk. Find out beforehand if her choice to feed the baby is breastfeeding. Offer to bring a meal the day you visit. Offer to help in whatever way without her listing the things she needs help with. If you own a home, you would understand the things that could bring comfort to someone in their time of need

Rest is vital and, therefore, be mindful of how long you keep a postpartum person awake during visits. Time yourselves when you visit and be sure not to overstay your welcome. Be mindful of advice and unsolicited tips unless they asked for advice and let them learn through their own mistakes. The newborn baby will be a baby for a long time. Let them rest in these first days because a time will come when they would ask for advice and you would then share.

Be patient with them. They are between the realms of life and death, and in the immediate postpartum. They are somewhere between losing their minds with all the information conveyed to them, all the planning that needs to be planned at home for the other children (if there are any), and finding their own souls. It is a process that nobody can really understand at face value. Do not believe what you see when you see her even, just know she is fighting so many battles within herself. If she shares them depends on the relationship you have with her.

Maybe start by asking

1. How was their birth experience? How did the partner experience it?
2. Is the baby healthy?
3. Is mama healthy and recovering well?
4. Did the baby come with health issues? How can you help them from now on?
5. Did the baby have to remain in the hospital?
6. Did the baby make it home?

7. How are the other children coping with an addition in the house?
8. How can you help to give the other child (ren) attention when the parents cannot?
9. What else would the family like to share
10. Be the friend that sticks around. Abandonment in grief is real

Being mindful of such details enables you to know the support the family needs. Not all babies come home, and a healthy baby is not true nor a given for many families. Before you even set foot to support check and understand how the birth was. If the baby came home and is healthy, be aware that they still need the time to find their own balance as a family and therefore if your presence is not helpful, maybe stay away until you can be useful.

Sometimes life happens when the baby remains in the hospital for whatever reason. Sometimes life simply starts in NICU. Be mindful that there will be a degree of grieving for the parents because they have lost the expectations of their dreams. Losing a beautiful birth experience because you, as a guest and even as a father, mother or sister-in-law, would not know if this was their last child and or if they can relive that experience again.

Sometimes babies may go home because they are stable enough even if life is not viable or will never be of quality to them. Many times these babies would go with tubes attached to them so that the parents can allow them to enjoy being home with their families. Many, even if it is known will not live, are given the chance to connect with their children in a home setting as long as they are explained the care part or with a home nurse.

Palliative care babies come with a lot of worry for the parents and often many grieve the loss of their perfect children. Many go through shame wondering in their own minds; *'was it their fault*? What is everyone thinking of me? Why couldn't we have a normal child like everyone else'. There are many things that are going on in these moments that go unnoticed and are not acknowledged. Because their own minds are racing with everything else, even for the grieving parents, sitting down to explain how they feel is a big puzzle and one that they cannot explain.

HOW CAN YOU SUPPORT THESE INSTANCES?

1. Support by allowing them to feel everything they are feeling
2. Listen to them vent or cry without judgment
3. Acknowledge that their emotions will be up and down
4. Take nothing that is shared or said in these moments personal
5. Validate their feelings, hurt, and disappointments too
6. Encourage them; nothing that happened was their fault
7. Be a part of the tapestry as it develops, because every part contributes to how the final work will become
8. Be like the children
9. Call them by name
10. Listen to understand

Grief is a long road that becomes a part of people's lives. Everyone has been affected, even the extended family. The focus is on the parents though and the siblings, if there are any. There are many decisions that have to be made by the parents, which unfortunately weigh on their hearts. There is so much denial, shock, pointing fingers, blame, shame, regret, and bargaining that happens regardless of how the birth developed. Be mindful and gentle.

Kissing: It is very dangerous to kiss a newborn baby because they are very fragile and can catch anything. Make a habit to kiss their little feet from now on. There are many sicknesses that lie low for a long time which can be very dangerous if a newborn baby whose immune system hasn't been built up yet. Herpes or mouth ulcers are one of those

1. **Hygiene** is very important, too. Be sure to wash your hands before touching anything that is linked to the baby and regularly, too. Sterilize your hands regularly until you can use water and soap to wash thoroughly. Babies have a very low and risky immune system, meaning they can become sick quickly.
2. **Allowing them to feel everything** is something that is hard for many parents to do. There is a doubt that creeps in that leave them feeling like they have to put on a front or a show and act as if they have it together. Let us not forget ancestral backgrounds also, especially in many indigenous cultures and African cultures where boys are raised to be strong and not show emotion
3. **Listen to them vent** many times. Parents feel judged for how they feel in the moment. You do not need to add or subtract anything from what they are sharing. Often, just your presence is enough
4. **Acknowledge that their emotions** would be up and down - there may be times you're around them they can hold a conversation and other times where they would rather just be alone without conversation. Availing yourself for both outcomes is important so that they can process things
5. **Take nothing said to you in these moments personally**. It may be someone snaps at you because they are so ragged and overwhelmed that even a 'simple' answer becomes a difficult thing to deliver. In these moments, they are not thinking rationally and are very sure there will be apologies coming your way when everything settles
6. **Validate their pain** - Listening to someone vent helps them feel heard where they probably were not listened to before. Being heard and listened to brings a feeling of being seen. If you

add nothing to the conversation, just being there and supporting them as they hurt and through their disappointments can be vital

7. **Encourage them** - that nothing that happened was their fault. Many times, this is one thing that eats the parents away, if they did anything or could have done anything to prevent what happened to their babies. The grief breaks people. It breaks families. Grief makes everyone a suspect, too. So often, they would look for who did what and who didn't do what.

8. **Be like children** - They really understand little, but they comprehend more than we give them credit. Many times, you will hear someone sharing how their children didn't have words. All they did was to be present, allowed their mother to cry, and comforted them with a hug or just by being in the space with them. I often say, when death happens in a family, a dark cloud sets in. Sometimes, through the fog of that cloud, the brain is not clear about what it really is seeing and what it is not. Many people even doubt their own shadows. By you being present, you allow the bereaved families to connect with their own senses at that moment in time. That they may realize, no, their mind is not playing with them, there really is someone with them holding space quietly

9. If there was already a name given to the baby who has died, **call them by their name**. Hearing the names called out louder validates their existence

10. **Listening is a skill not everyone has**. Many times, people listen to respond. Make a habit of listening to understand than to answer. Many people hear what needs to be responded to and miss the point completely. Show up authentically, if at all, especially in these sacred spaces. Showing up and being present for people authentically means listening to understand. Listening to be present. Listening allows the other person to be heard. Not everything said or spoken out loudly demands an answer or justification

11. **Photography:** Ask before you take pictures of someone's baby, even if it is your grandchild. Ancestrally, the face of the baby was never plastered everywhere for all sundry to see it. The same protection that was shown to the newborn mother or birthing person was extended to the baby because spiritually, we say, 'every energy that is negative attracts to all that is pure. Newborn babies are pure souls, hence the protection to share so much about them with the outside world and too soon too. It is a choice, but protect your lineage, because you can

Also, be mindful of these two terms; Postpartum Depression and Postpartum period. Many people confuse or associate postpartum with depression, and that is not true. In fact, the postpartum is the most tranquil moment in any person's life during the childbearing years because back home, the family gathered together in strong unity to support you through this RITE of passage because of the returning ancestor but also because there is a traditional and cultural belief that childbirth is risky and can be fatal and therefore; it is not a given to survive childbirth.

In the western world, the postpartum period is associated with misery, struggling parents, dysfunctional homes, and struggle. Pregnancy, Birth, and Postpartum is an industry that is growing more than rapidly with tones of appropriation and revamping of other people's cultures. And therefore, it is very clear that the narrative of struggle and looking for fixes benefits someone.

Products that could almost open a home pharmacy are flung left, right and center, and instead of people seeking knowledge from within, you find many first-time parents jumping at every 'solution' proposed out there because suddenly it is not normal for a newborn baby to cry and guaranteed there is a bottle of fix that can help them.

Many still describe **postpartum** as **depression**. Someone would want to express their experience but explains it as 'I also had that postpartum, it was a nightmare. Postpartum means **'after birth'**. It is **the period after birth.** Postpartum depression is depression that happens during the Postpartum Period. However; depression can already be present before pregnancy and during pregnancy.

Ancestrally, this is a moment to thrive as a family and build strong roots of togetherness, support, community, and the true village. Back in Africa, a 'village' is inclusive and bears more meaning than simply a collection. It is the close-knit understanding of how we need each other to thrive and raise the next generations with virtues and knowledge that they may keep for the generation to come. The elderly looked at the growth of the young and the young generation looked upon the older generation for the wisdom they have accumulated and the stories of resilience, strength, and co-existing together that have happened since the beginning of time amongst our people

One can be depressed before and during the pregnancy, and that depression can then continue into the postpartum period. Labor outcomes can experience during labor itself and can also trigger depression. We need to be mindful when we interchange these two words:

(1) Depression is a term on its own and so is **(2)** Postpartum Depression.

There are many other perinatal mood and anxiety disorders that can develop beyond postpartum depression, which either never were present, to begin with, or develop immediately and as time progresses, like

1. Postpartum PTSD (Post-traumatic Stress Disorder)

2. Postpartum OCD (Postpartum Obsessive-Compulsive Disorder)
3. Postpartum Depression & Anxiety

> *Everyone wants to hold the baby, but who holds the parents? Ancestrally, they say it takes a village to raise a child and the same village to raise competent and resilient parents too - Naomie Karemi KAINGU*

News of a newborn baby gets everyone in excitement immediately. For many, though, the thought of checking in on the birthing person or the mother (she/her) does not come naturally. There is something about a baby's arrival that perks up excitement in forgetting the 'main character' in the whole 'show', the parent. The focus continues to be on the bump and on babies that make it to go home safe and sound and healthy, too. The focus remains on plan A, where everything works out fine and the whole family unit makes it back home until that does not happen.

In my native country Kenya, this news is usually not shared with the outside world even, because the focus is not only on the baby but on the mother returning from her journey of birth. Natively, it is something that we realize and that is part of the reason her postpartum period would start at eight months of pregnancy and not after 8 weeks.

It is from her eighth month that the expectant couple would pack up and go back to their own parent's home or the in-laws to prepare for the birth. It is understood that in the eighth month they would slow down, and therefore their brain capacity is also slower. She is more forgetful and needs to connect with her womb and baby in readiness. There are rituals and ceremonies performed when they return home to prepare for the birth because, culturally, we believe every new baby within a homestead is an ancestor returning.

There is the belief that they have come for a purpose and therefore we honor the person who not only carried them for 9 months, but also nurtured them, and then birthed them. In Africa as a continent, we keep family names and therefore, this returning ancestor has to be protected come what may, reason their arrival is never shared far and beyond until they have passed the **'sabaa'** the seventh day after birth and then the extended family does not even hold the baby until they have concluded their 40th-day celebration.

So! According to everyone else, everything at the birth went well. That may not be true, but following me a bit here. There is a new addition in the friends' circle and everyone wants to come on over and hold the new addition to the family. Everyone wants to come and be acquainted with the new baby, but what about the newborn parents? The mother (she/her) who birthed? What about her aches and pains? Is anyone interested in meeting the new version of them? Is anyone interested in whether the bruising is 'down there and how the swelling might treat her? There is more than meets the eye and a perfect new mother is not one of them.

There are many struggles that are not written on the foreheads of a newborn mother or birthing person. Our duty as caregivers and support workers is to be mindful of the energies we bring into these spaces. We walk into spaces that are very open and fragile, and many times people have still not landed regardless of how the birth developed. In my line of work, I use three elements as a guide for myself to make sure I am filling up their cups as new parents going through all the sleepless nights and the initial worries and not adding on to the stress. I use the terms HUG before I head out to visit my postpartum families (the families I am supporting)

Many times when you walk into the space of immediate birth and bereavement, it is to realize and acknowledge that things are not like you imagine them to be. That they may put on a front because they do not want to disturb you or come across as weak and it is easier to act like it is all good when deep down it is not. Society has added a significant load of guilt and shame on birthing people's backs from the moment there is a positive test. There are expectations you would manage without fail and everything can be fixed, too. Women are good at covering up and accumulating a lot because of a lot of things. The younger generation is even harder to work with because they reign from a quick-fix era.

They expect to queue up at McDonald's the following day after childbirth because then everyone in their circles will know they are strong and not whiney. Many times when being coached or supported, it can be very difficult to get past someone who is over-informed with the wrong information, though. Sometimes it is what society has enabled to brain-feed us that perfection in parenting exists, other times it is the fear of being judged and then there is the guilt of feeling inadequate and incapable when it should come naturally, whatever natural means.

Be mindful of what comes to you immediately, and what you utter. Going in and exclaiming at someone '***you are looking good***' would really shut them down from within, even though they would never say it to your face.

> *The postpartum period is an extension of pregnancy and birth. It is not the end. Naomie Karemi KAINGU.*

The danger of spouting statements like that to someone who has not revealed if they really are feeling good about themselves is; that you will end up muting them. Once you say that to someone who is struggling internally without letting the world know she is, would stop them from being honest with you when they probably should have been honest. You saying those words takes away her need to be vulnerable, which is probably what she needed to do. *'You said I look good. How dare I tell you differently?'*

As birth workers and the support system, we must collectively be mindful of the emotions at hand and the need to share our own versions of joys. Being mindful of our own **positive stories** when we walk into these spaces is vital. Many times, they are not ready to process anything else from outside because they are going through their own struggles and adjusting as a family. And mostly, they are not ready to hear it because *'**they have not landed**'*

Indigenously women were looked after by their lineage of women and the men could go nowhere near them so sex was not something that was done before the 40-day celebration was concluded and that's part of the reason you will be pampered and prepared like the bride because now after that 40 days you're going back to your marital home, not only as a mother but as a mother and a wife so you can continue from where you left off.

This is part of the reason in Africa as a continent, the postpartum is not six and eight weeks. Postpartum **is eternal** because there will never be another version of your pre-birth. There will be many versions of you staying on the roll from the moment your baby is born. For many, the forgetfulness that pregnancy gifted them will take a very long time to combat. Many complain of hips or joint pains 3/4 years after birth. The body changes to accustom to the new you and with that come different struggles, adjustments, acceptance, and joy too.

Six and eight weeks postpartum is what we know in the first world and even then, the mother is never the center of conversation unless it is about contraception and when she is not 'allowed' to get pregnant again based on whether she birthed surgically. Many of them, by the time the 8 weeks check-up comes along, feel more 'human' so for those who know how to, the nearness and the made-up faces hide their struggles really well.

Back home, news of the baby means the extended family is to prepare for the 40th-day celebration and will allow that family to adjust without pressure. Everyone who should know is aware that the baby has arrived, and the support you would normally get is loved ones bringing you meals but never stepping foot inside the home because everyone understands how tough those first weeks of birth are. People will support you from a distance. Africans, as a people, love our prints. This would be incorporated with you and then the print will be chosen for the big day. It is very customary for family members to dress in the same pattern so that well-wishers can identify them within the gathering and offer their congratulations as needed.

Parenting is naturally isolating and lonely. There are many clouds that set in when a baby is born. Often, the friend lists go down because the timeline and responsibilities of a baby take over. Your availability is another factor where the baby's need and priority come first; you are tired of keeping up with the extended nightlife that you once could do Monday to Monday. There is the need for safety and trust in who you are leaving your baby with, and so much more. Then there is the fear of how others perceive you as a parent

> **HUG** stands for **H** for **Help,** **U** for **Understanding, and G** for **Guidance**

SETTING UP SUPPORT - IMMEDIATE NETWORK

Many hide their struggles for fear of being judged. Many don't know if their choices will be received well on their own. As women, especially the older generation, we need to look at our own biases too because the '*medals of motherhood*' is what makes young mothers struggle in silence. There is no one way to raise a family and therefore how you raised children in 1979 will never be how children will be raised in 2023, for example.

The notion that 'I did it so get on with it can be very harmful when young parents are faking things in order to match up to their seniors because of the fear of coming across as weak, incapable, and 'what will the world say if I say I am struggling. Parent shaming is another one that is rife, especially with the extended and in-laws. Just because they struggled does not mean you should. Nobody else's normal will be yours either. This actually brings nothing but shame and negative attention to something that many of the older generations deem 'normal'.

Children of this newer generation demand a lot of attention and focus, not like the ones from the 80s, for example. Parents these days both work more than full-time jobs to provide a decent way of life for their families. The cost of living is nowhere near what it was back in 1970 either, I am sure and therefore people need to show up and stand tall to be seen in society.

In the western world, we could still try to support where we can meaningfully. There are websites that help create online calendars where loved ones and those who are available to support can sign up, choose a date, and state the support they can provide.

One website I love is **www.mealtrain.com** because, with this system, everyone sees who picked what date and what they would do for the family and they can then plan themselves accordingly

The benefit of the meal train is that in not so many ways, it holds people accountable. Once you have assigned yourself a day to do whatever, it becomes disappointing to cancel your commitment, knowing the family relied on your support. Also, it enables everyone involved to choose what, how, and when they can support you based on what has already been offered.

What can you do to help the family settle in calmly?

1. Bring soup with you on your way to them
2. If you are not well health-wise, do not visit. Newborn babies are prone to catch anything that goes, be mindful
3. You can help them batch cook and freeze ready-to-eat meals
4. Help them with childcare of the other children (if there are any)
5. Help them with the housework that needs to be done
6. Acknowledge that sleep is a pillar in recovery, so let them sleep whenever they need to!
7. See what needs doing without asking (many times they would retaliate and put a front)
8. Help them with steaming their bodies if they choose to

Soup - Everybody can make soup. Some people can't, but these days many supermarkets stock the most delicious soups that you can take to a family to nourish them.

Self-check - Babies catch everything that is going on. If you are not well health-wise, maybe defer an appointment to see the baby until you feel well. If you have children and are planning to take everyone with you, the same applies to everybody. Chickenpox is one that can damage even for a pregnant person and even if the blisters gave popped and they show no symptoms or complaints anymore, please defer until everyone is well enough.

Batch cook - There are many meals that you can make ahead of time and freeze even cupcakes and muffins so that they are ready to warm and serve. Food like Quiche keep longer in the fridge and are great for offering a cup of soup. As the time of birth progresses and you want to help prepare them for the long nights and unrested days, organize an afternoon of togetherness and help them batch cook.

Offer to look after the other children - When a newborn mother arrives home, it is in her nature to want to look after the other children even when she is exhausted and not able to. If you are around, you could either look after them at home or offer to take them away so that they can also get a distraction that is fun and the attention they cannot get immediately, because there is a lot that may go on in her head at that moment whilst she finds her own ground and calm. Realize that for many, time to adjust is vital. If they do eventually, they can prosper as a family.

Everyone can clean too - You don't have to go in and turn the place upside down in the name of cleaning. If you make the areas where she would use tidy and calm for her, that would already be something. The toilet she would use is important, as the surfaces she would touch because she would then touch her newborn baby. There is also something calming that a clean home brings, even through turmoil.

Acknowledge that sleep is a pillar - in recovery. Allow them to rest and catch up on the broken sleep, which is the norm in the first weeks. Don't overstay your visit and if you do, get busy elsewhere while she catches a sleep maybe by getting her tray ready for when she is up, making by making chai ready in the thermos, sterilizing the bottle/pacifiers if the baby is using them, you could help sterilize the breastfeeding kit because these are the little jobs that add up and cause the biggest stress is the first weeks of parenting.

See what else needs doing - without being asked. Many times they would act like they have to be all under control, but no Womb-man went through this RITE of passage alone. We have always had family gather around and rightfully, the extra hand makes for a calm transition. So do without being asked because they will never ask and do not accept a random 'we are good. You could help with putting laundry in the washing machine too. There are many areas you could help a newborn family with, and without being in their faces.

Help her with steaming - if she chooses it. Steaming the body once the flow reduces is such a treat. It has many benefits and requires some preparation. If she wants to do that, you could help set the steaming chair in the bathroom for her, boil the herbs that would be needed and get everything she would need near. Somebody would need to hold the baby if they are awake, and that would be your moment to get in close with cuddles and let her enjoy the moment of the throne. It can be an emotional moment because many women relive the moments of their births and therefore be on guard that she would need you completely

Nine

IF IT DOES NOT SOUND RIGHT, DO NOT SAY IT

As much as we would like for all pregnancy journeys to end with babies who make it home, it is not a reality for many parents. Not all babies get to go home, that is a fact, unfortunately. Please hold on to this paragraph, whilst you continue reading…

As family members and the immediate support network, being mindful of the words we utter are vital. Be mindful of your 'happy positive' experiences that you cannot wait to exchange notes and have others hear it because it is not the place for it nor is it a nice thing to do when someone is adjusting, going through a difficult postpartum phase and even more so, where the baby did not get to come home.

Understandably, death is a taboo topic, especially when it is the death of a child. People tend to 'hush-hush' around this taboo topic, even those we deem close to us. The stillness that death portrays is what scares people and shuts them from being normal around it, regardless of how many deaths they have witnessed throughout their lives.

Therefore; the 'need' to help and make the situation less painful is one that makes people say the wrong things or things that may seem very insensitive at the worst time. Many feel the 'need to be or do something to 'ease' the pain of the bereaved parents, not realizing that many times it is not the words that comfort a bereaved parent but the presence that they were not left alone that makes them feel held, without words, without discussions and simply by others being present in their space. Their minds are so busy that sometimes all they need is assurance that they are not losing their minds by imagining that they are in the presence of others.

> *One thing bereaved parents struggle with is feeling ashamed after losing a child. Naomie Karemi KAINGU.*

Many times, people want to help, but they simply do not know how. If you are in doubt, though of what help is needed within a family setting, simply ask. Often, though, you would be met with retaliation of some sort because asking for help and accepting it is something that African people have issues dealing with it. I am the same. I love having people around, cooking, and being merry with everyone, but the moment someone says 'next time come to mine' it becomes something that I feel my legs heavily lifting me.

I dislike putting pressure on or disturbing people, and therefore I keep a lot to myself. I am learning to let go though, because the village will only come forth when they know where they can be present. If what is at the tip of your tongue leaves you feeling like maybe you should not say it, don't. As a mother who has experienced loss before, I use this guide. I often think about what I wanted someone to say to me. I often go back and think about what I wanted someone to read between the lines to support us.

> *The postpartum period back home is eternal. Not 6 and 8 weeks like we are made to see and believe - Naomie Karemi KAINGU.*

So whilst they are in the early moments of their postpartum recovery, availing themselves is one part many people struggle with. Remember, unless you offer it sternly, they would always say 'they have things in control' so many times I say just do it (whatever that may be) and apologize later if that is not how they do it themselves. Nobody likes a dirty home, and cleaning is something that everyone can do. If you can, avail yourself to make sure the simplest cleaning duties are done. If you are unsure, ask.

Everybody handles loss differently, but you can not assume that they are dealing with things just because they look calm and collected. Whatever you think may go on, best keep it to yourself, and observe where you think they may need support and offer it without prejudice or judgment. I say this because even I was not exempt from the judgments back in the day when our second child arrived and my parents-in-law assumed because I was discharged from the hospital I should have been ready.

Judgments were pouring from every visit and how I couldn't keep up with xyz.. forgetting the birth I had had, and the diagnosis we had received. Cleaning the house sparkling clean before your arrival will not be that new parent's priority.

Their priority in every postpartum phase is to find balance and strength, not serve or host you. Making sure the house is spot on before you arrive is not ok either. This narrative needs to change because if you have carried life yourself and went through this phase, relive those moments when you wished someone would come and help you, and because you did not need or get that support, does not mean someone else does not need it.

As women, mothers and parents, we need to stop being so judgemental and sit on our biases sometimes. Just because you could do it does not mean everybody can. Respect that every parent's struggle will be different compared to yours. Not everyone gets the pleasure of saying their pregnancy journey or the births of their babies were magnificent.

Romanticizing pregnancies and birth experiences can be quite harmful because experiences differ in subsequent pregnancies and also among families.

The need for others to see you as mother-of-all-mothers, the 'strong mama' within the group, and coming out all heavy with your parenthood medals is sometimes unreal and very unhelpful. It can be very damaging too. If you find it dirty and see the need for it to be cleaned, do it or leave it as is.

When you walk into a home with new parents and you see something that needs doing, do it but don't, then sit them down and explain what you did and how they should do it. This is rife with the in-laws and it is one that needs to be capped because everybody's challenges and struggles are different.

Keep judgment away if you will help otherwise stay away because your judgment is not what the family needs in their moment of restructuring, re-grounding or xyz.

> *There is no medal for the best pregnancy journey or birth experience. Naomie Karemi KAINGU*

This one is a hint for the partners; as a father or partner, you know what your own side of the family is like towards your wife or partner. As much as we would love for families to have close-knit relations, that unfortunately is not a reality for many. So if you know your side of the family is heavy with judgments, try to buy time until she can stomach it.

These are the things that break relationships because when she is in her deepest dump going through emotions and feelings and someone comes with a biting judgemental comment in the name of 'complimenting' or 'advise' which usually is unsolicited, it can be very hurtful and is for many times, it remains hurtful for a long time because an expectant person and when they are in their postpartum phase is something many never forget for a very long time.

This is the moment she will never forget how she was made to feel when she was at her worst. Be her protector whilst she is trying to balance recovering and continuing being the wife she was before childbirth and maintaining a family relation too with the in-laws. Stand up for her at the moment when she would have to defend her decisions as a mother and parent to your child/ren because parenting like pregnancy invites unwanted and unwarranted advice or comments when you least expect it.

If there is news of another pregnancy, it may be better for the news to come directly from the person bearing the news i.e. the sister/sister-in-law instead of someone else as this may be perceived as hearsay but also remember that though it is not anyone else's responsibility to carry and bear the pain of the bereaved, being sensitive to how that news will make them 'feel' is kind.

Please also remember that she/he may not be extremely joyful for you immediately or there may be some kind of awkwardness depending on how long their baby/child died.

Ten

EMPTY HANDS, FULL BREASTS

Unfortunately, as much as we would all love to have babies come home, not all of them get to go home. It is a sad reality, but what remains hopeful is that people will speak about their experiences and share their stories of their babies who came but did not stay. The aspect that loss is part of childbirth was included in the teachings within the community.

There is an understanding that the babies choose their families and sometimes they just don't get to accomplish the connection, but spiritually their souls try until they accomplish it. There are stories shared where a couple lost 2 or 3 babies until the 4th living child came and they would sometimes reveal that they tried to connect with the family three times before, but it was not possible.

The education that pregnancy does not conclude is shared because either way, the clan would give thanks for the possibility of having had the lineage extended and therefore the expectant couple would still thank the ancestors whilst they waited to be blessed. Gratitude is practiced in all outcomes.

Part of the reason was that because news of the pregnancy was shared with a very close-knit group of people, should the pregnancy change course, the same level of support was available to you throughout. It is very unfortunate when a pregnancy ends without a living child whether they were born still or did not stay long and a pregnancy ended with a miscarriage. Support at this moment is vital for everyone around the expectant couple. Bereavement is a taboo topic even amongst the older generation because babies who did not live were treated differently and many of the older generations would attest to the fact that many were not given the opportunity to see their babies or view them before they were taken away.

Bereavement is one aspect that still leaves people 'drawing blanks' in how they can be helpful to a friend, relative, or colleague who has experienced the death of their baby. Human nature is that we want to help and fix things when they are broken. When there is news of a baby's death as humans, we want to help the bereaved parents. Trying to help them cope or feel our presence in support.

What is actually needed at the moment of grieving is simply for others to be a part of their grieving process. You do not need to fix anything because nothing can be fixed. Simply be around a bereaved couple or parents. Repeatedly, the words I hear from bereaved parents are that it helped to have someone with them to help plan things. A lot needs to happen in a very short period following the death of a baby, and it helps to have someone help to slow down the pace. Too much needs to be agreed upon, ticked, and signed for all whilst you are coming to terms with the fact that your baby is no more.

By about day three, four, and for some people on day five, the milk supply doubles slowly bringing with it a lot of emotions because the increase demands a lot from a newborn mother energy-wise but also with a living baby the sucking reflex normally changes because with an increase in milk the latch is different, baby does not drink enough to empty the breasts or some babies feed more frequently too. This is the moment they call engorgement. For some, it can bring fever and emotional turmoil because the hormones are already all over the place but the sudden lack of a minute to breathe can be emotional because it would appear all you do is feed, clean bottles, feed, and change the baby. The repetitive work can be a trigger for some people

WHEN THE OUTCOME IS HEAVIER THAN YOU IMAGINED

And It would be... hold on to the people who stick around to help you through it. Hold on to the people who do not keep you in the pity pit where they offer nothing more than pity for your situation. That kind of support will keep you in that pit of misery for longer than you wish to be in it. Surround yourself with people who will notice the darkness of the pit you are in, and offer you their hand to help pull you out. They do not have to promise anything or say much, but simply showing they are available to you so you are not going through the phase of trial alone is enough to help you along the way. It will not be easy, but with the right support, you will learn and grow from your experience.

Be mindful of the energy you welcome at this moment, because the people you need around you are those who will help you see the beauty of the event. Hard as it may be, sometimes we have to show up even when we are broken to continue. You do not have to pretend that it does not hurt, that it did not shake you to your core, or that it does not sting however many years later, but don't stay in that moment forever. Experiences come to teach us about our resilience, our strength, and even our capabilities. Give yourself patience, be gentle with yourself, and embrace yourself with grace first and the rest will follow around you. Remember that energies attract what is present.

WHATEVER YOU DO

Eat first. In your grief, you may dismiss your need for energy and your mental load will be clogged for quite a while as well. What will help you stay afloat is food. Food will help your mental capacity remain optimum.

You will think clearly at some point and decide for your little one and family that matter. If you are a family member, friend, or colleague supporting a family through bereavement, please be patient with them. They may refuse the first plate, the first cups of tea, but don't stop offering them though and being supportive. They might say no to begin with, but over time accept it because their bodies will demand it as well.

Your arms being empty is the hardest, regardless of how long you carried the life you did. What you have lost is your future, not your today, and hurts. Nothing will ever be the same again. Family dynamics might also change and the gap may take a lifetime to fill up. Typically, your body will start producing milk by around day 3 or 4 with a full-term loss, and that may hit you harder. What you could do if you are not planning to donate your milk to another child or your local NICU (Neonatal Intensive Care Unit) is start wearing a tight bra before your birth. Gravity and stimulation help bring milk in. By wearing a tight bra, you tell the body that milk production is not needed.

You will need to wear a tight bra even under the shower because warm water may stimulate your glands. Speak to your midwife also for medication options. Sometimes you will need medication to stop your milk production by prescription. There are herbs also that you could use like Sage, which helps with overproduction, Oregano, which could be used in cooking, can help equalize overproduction and stop production altogether. Kale is one that is almost forgotten in the category of 'do not consume' during postpartum, but Kale can really stop milk production. The last one is Parsley. Beautiful aroma and a lovely spice to add to curries but large amounts have been found to influence milk production. You could also have loads of cups of fresh Mint tea.

LOOK AFTER YOURSELF

Ancestrally, a woman (She/Her) who lost a child either by miscarriage or stillbirth was taken care of by her elders.

What they did was massage her and introduce heat to her body using warmed-up khangas so that she released whatever energies she was holding on to. She was rubbed down with warmed towels to relieve body aches and treated as a postpartum person. She got everything done for her as if her baby lived because she carried life.

With the body wraps, words were spoken and prayers were offered, so she held on to the memory of her child. Prayers were offered to the ancestors gone before to receive the child in an embrace. The woman is then wrapped from head to toe to create a cocoon where she can release her emotions and embrace the feeling of being held. She would be encouraged to pray for her departed child's soul and still give thanks to her body for having received the egg and nurture it because by giving thanks, traditionally it is believed that the souls of the next children will pick you again and the gods of fertility will bless a grateful heart to wipe your tears.

She is then encouraged to bound every day for the comfort binding brings. Binding the belly gives you a supported feeling, helps keep your belly area warm, helps with post-cramps, and also helps you recover quicker. Your blood loss is more, but within a short period, you can start steaming with warm water placed under an open seat to help you release anything that needs to be released and cleanse your womb too. And then, in the same way as the celebration of a living baby, she is honored and celebrated back into the community as they go back to burial and say their goodbyes to their departed baby being supported throughout. Sometimes the storms will be silent and other times they would be so loud you won't hear yourselves think. Be comforted that it is ok to feel whatever it is you would be feeling, allow yourselves to feel them.

> **Your feelings are valid and you may feel it all. - Naomie Karemi KAINGU**

For family, friends, and colleagues: The one thing that is so important at this moment is the support of others. Do not ask what they need, speak to the immediate family members and come up with a supporting plan that will ensure that after everyone is gone and life has gone back for everyone else, this couple is supported through that first moment of isolation so that they do not fall into depression and emotional turmoil alone. The first moments of being alone after a baby's death can confuse, confirming.

Realize that often, one cannot let go of situations that made them sad, because they were also the events that made them happy. People rejoice at the sound of pregnancy and the thought of a newborn baby coming amongst them. It is devastating when this does not come to fruition. Understand that this kind of void one never really gets over it. Mourn with them, avail and support them where you can.

Eleven

HONOUR YOUR POSTPARTUM

Regardless of the length, you carried life because

> *Postpartum is for EVERY womb that has carried life™ - Naomie Karemi KAINGU*

Whether a baby lives to go home, there is a level of grief that happens with childbirth that is unexplainable. Childbirth takes away a part of your being and replaces it with another, and the part that departs can remain like a cloud for many people whilst they try to understand what actually happened.

Honoring your postpartum period is vital with the right support so that you can learn from what others will share, from the pictures they allow you to see, and from the stories that will be shared in your midst.

Honor your postpartum so that you may 'arrive' in the new version of yourself. Many people who are attuned spiritually will attest that there is a level of wandering that happens in the immediate postpartum whilst you are trying to make sense of what happened, but also the next steps ahead. It is not surprising that following the birth of a baby there is a lost gaze that is clear in the birthing person's eyes and many times they do not look anyone in the eyes no matter how long they were present with them before the baby was born. This wandering explains why that 'golden hour' is important not only for bonding but also for the soul to settle.

This is part of the reason newborn mothers (She/Her) were left to recover before everyone came their way. They were attended to in a calm and patient manner because this moment needs supportive people to help slow the pace and bring calm within a family unit that is adjusting mentally, emotionally, and spiritually too. Nobody expected to turn up and find her all made up because she needed time to 'land' and expecting that of anybody who has just given birth currently is not only inconsiderate, it is very insensitive.

Especially for the parents who have gone to lose babies in any stage of their childbearing years, the wombs that carried babies who did not stay, you are just as much in the postpartum period as anybody else is. Do not overlook your need for rest and your need to take things slowly because your body went through the same process of receiving, nurturing, and growing in life. The time that life grew in your womb is irrelevant.

> *I say, 'the postpartum is for every womb that has carried life™*
> *- Naomie Karemi KAINGU*

Even though your baby didn't get to come home and regardless of whether they stayed in your womb for 3-4 weeks, or were born asleep. And therefore, is calm and concluded, please honor your postpartum period, process what needs processing, and give your baby a name even if it is a nickname because naming them validates their existence and will help you with identifying that void and your grieving process with a name behind it. It will give your process a different feeling also as you associate it with a name. Please give yourself grace through the process because it is not a journey for the faint-hearted.

Allow yourself to recover from carrying that life. If you allow yourself to realign with your hormones, your body will adjust to it. Take the time to listen to your own heartbeat. If a decision had to be made, that was not your choice but a 'must'. Remember that the choice you made was the right one for you and your family. Never second-guess yourself.

It will help with your recovery if you slow down. Slowing down will help you get back into your routines and functioning. Slowing down will help you with self-discovery after all the turmoil is calmed down, and you need to love yourself to continue loving those around you.

Grief is heavy. It is a journey with no expiry date. A journey that is isolating and lonely. One that even when you are surrounded by people is isolating because few understand the gap or pain one feels unless they have experienced the same pain. It is one void that to understand it, have to have lived it as well.

So it can be quite complicated even for those we love dear to understand sometimes. A moment would show up when you could speak about your loss without breaking down, but that comes in time. The notion that you get better at it is another aspect of bereavement support that is baffling.

> **Nobody and nothing gets better at grieving.** *You simply learn to cope and maneuver around it. - Naomie Karemi KAINGU*

The number of children you will have following your loss will never replace the child you lost. Because of the fear of losing another child, subsequent pregnancies may be more difficult. The hope to achieve certain milestones will be present and, therefore, memories of your baby who died can come back to the surface.

The presence of your next baby after loss will certainly wipe your tears, but you will hurt. Grief will always be present, even when you will parent your next baby. Take all the moments that trigger you as they are, identify them, and try to avoid them if you can

Twelve

HONOR YOUR POSTPARTUM - SPLIT

HOW CAN YOU SUPPORT HER AS A PARTNER?

As a partner, you may deal with your own sorrow and shock, but because you are the 'head of the family, you try to keep this 'ship sailing'. Don't forget yourself too through the processing. You also need to process things and find your inner peace to support her through it. You could try to speak when you are both calm, to find out where you both are in your journey of grief.

Recognize that she may close and stay within herself, maybe simply shut down, lash out and maybe be completely silent while she processes everything quietly. Do not make her feel like she should be any other way. As her immediate support system, realize that you will not understand a lot of what is going on in her head. There may be days when she will speak about things and get very emotional, other days she would not want to talk about it, and other times she may talk like she is calm. Be aware that her emotions will be up and down.

Please also remember that support starts from within before it is sourced outside. You can hire people to come in and support you, but these people will only be in your home for 6-8 hours in the day. For the rest of the hours, those within the home need to know how to support her and let her feel like she can have all the feelings without being judged. Because you know her limits and what she normally is like, I would explain to your immediate folk to be mindful to avoid incidents.

Be aware also that she may just be fine going through whatever she may be going through and wanting to do the 'normal' things, too. Doing things helps distract some people and if this is her way of dealing with things, support her through it. Family and friends supporting in these moments need to be mindful of the 'advice' and well wishes or words said in good faith that can cut deeper than they imagine. I am sure you have heard so many examples already, but one that comes to mind is '**they are in a better place**.

Now anyone who thinks a baby's '*better place* is in the grave and not its mother's arms need not be anywhere near a bereaved parent/family. These kinds of 'well-meant' lines can be very damaging if only we are vigilant and careful about using them in the rawest and most heavy moments of people's lives. Naturally, death is scary and many people, even those near us, are never sure what to say. There are a lot of uncertainties and tiptoeing that happen when an event such as the death of a child happens.

People are afraid of saying the wrong things, and they inevitably end up saying exactly the wrong things. Well! at least you can have another one is one that is thrown around a lot where parents have lost babies. Having other children does not replace the ones parents have lost. In fact, the pregnancies following loss are the hardest for many reasons and they are filled with so much doubt, fear, and disbelief that they forget to connect with their bumps and enjoy the pregnancy journey because it is simply difficult.

For many families, these babies were prayed for and were very wanted. Parents don't connect with their babies only when they get to be born, strapped in a Maxi-Cosi, and make it home. **Parents connect with their babies the moment they test positive.** So the moment they see that extra line on the test strip, that is already somebody's future. Let us be mindful when we step foot in these spaces because they are very open, they are very emotional and you may end up saying the worst thing you can never take back and also ruin a long-term relationship just by thinking you are helping when actually you are causing more pain.

When we walk into this space, being mindful of what we say and how we say it too sometimes can be profound. You may be the only person who would step foot into that space that day who would make them feel supported. Thrive to be the person who brings comfort, leaving them feeling much better than they felt before you arrived, because your words may be the ones that save a life or create an impact on their lives at that moment or day.

Remember that for many, their struggles will never be on their forehead for all sundry to see. Many also know how to sweep things under the carpet until they become statistics where everyone thought they were coping until it is known shockingly that they were not. They will not burden their support network with their pain, disappointment, and anguish. Many would also do that to come across as strong. It's always the 'strong 'ones' that we need to pay even more attention to because they believe so much that they are in control that it becomes their reality until they flip.

Ask to join in on the journaling that you each write a page about how you are feeling at that moment. Sometimes it would feel like it's you against the world and other times you are against each other. Many couples find it so hard to share their pain with each other. Many men, especially, are better at texting than writing, so you may find if he is not in front of you, he will say what is really bothering him and how much it hurts more than he would in front of you.

Accept each other's way of dealing with things and validate each other's feelings. Listen to understand, not to answer.

HOW CAN YOU HOLD SPACE - AS A LOVED ONE OR A FRIEND?

For many people where the death of a child has happened or loss of any magnitude, many don't know how to be or if there is something they can do to help the family feel ok. There really is nothing anyone can do, not even for each other. There is also no way fits all that I will share with you, but there is one thing you can do that is so natural and will cause no one to feel a certain way. ***Just be***

They do not need you perfect, tip-toeing, and bringing awkwardness. Your presence and availability can make a huge change, one that you did not expect yourself. When you are present, be there to offer a listening ear and validate their pain. Listen to understand and offer compassion, not answer back. Be mindful of sharing your own experiences. Sometimes what you share may not be what they are looking for or helpful. Do not compare the feelings you felt, for example, when your pet died to what your friends are dealing with. *The death of a pet, sad as it is, is never comparable to the death of a baby.*

Many times, that is all that is needed. For many people who go through depression and grief, mental fog is something that comes up every time they speak up about how they felt in the moment and time. With the mental fog, sometimes they begin to doubt themselves and if what they see is true or they imagine it to be; 'was someone else sitting in the room with me, or was I imagining that? Companionship in grief is important because isolation can prolong how they recover and get up to continue also

If you are somebody who may say things out of the norm because you can't help it or are not comfortable saying 'nothing', maybe delegate yourself to tasks where you do not have to be in their presence per se but still get the things that need getting done from a distance. It may be arranging flowers for the ceremony or decorating their home or the venue for the ceremony, or looking after the rest of the children (if there are any) and cooking them a meal.

Keep the memory of your friend's child alive. Many forget after the ceremony is done, expecting the bereaved parents to 'get over it and continue living. Whilst continuing to live is something we must do and evidently have to, be mindful that grief is a journey and it does not get better after the burial is concluded. **Grief is a lifelong journey.** Although the bereaved family will seem to do better after their child's death, moments that are challenging come to them frequently.

Maybe from their own circle of friends or work colleagues, for example, who were expecting a baby or a pregnancy announcement. Triggers remain in their lives for always. As a friend, your best bet would be to avail yourself when the going gets heavy and when they need someone to talk to. Remember, you do not need to fix anything, be the listening ear and comforter. *'I know it is heavy and hard right now, but I am here to sit with you through it* is something that can bring so much comfort to a bereaved parent.

Another way you could help your friend process her grief is by holding a blessing ceremony, for example. Ancestrally women gathered because the collective of female energies, strategies, and visions have helped many African communities to prosper. Gathering everyone in honor of the baby for your friends will tell them you celebrate the fact that their baby came. Did not stay, but they came. **Honor the baby on this day by using their names.** Remember to ask everyone to mention the baby's name because it can be healing for the parents to know also why it is everyone has gathered and also for their own bodies to process the grieving period because of their child.

Parents do not connect with their babies only when they get to be strapped in a maxi-Cosi and make it home. Parents connect with their babies from the moment they test positive. Naomie Karemi KAINGU

HOW CAN YOU SUPPORT YOURSELF?

Realize that the Postpartum period is not difficult because you think you are failing at it. It is difficult because it is simply that - difficult. It can be very brutal than what you imagined it to be, pre-pregnant. So when your mother instincts hint to you that the pregnancy may become void, you can prepare ahead of time. When it is confirmed that you are going to have a loss, setting up your birth space is just as important. You can set up a warm bath for yourself, have some water to drink, and

1. Create a pace you can love on each other in
2. Forgive yourself and give yourself grace
3. Process the event
4. Belly Binding
5. Keeping warm
6. Allowing your body to rest
7. Eating nourishing warm food
8. Acknowledge your feelings
9. Talk to someone

10. Steaming and body works
11. Add warming herbs & spices to meals and drinks
12. Taking things slow
13. Creating a moment to speak to one another calmly
14. Give thanks
15. Journaling
16. Don't lose yourselves through the process
17. Choose your battles

Create a space you can call home. So that you can love each other in it - Where you can allow yourselves to feel without being judged. Where you can allow yourselves to be and hold each other's space privately as you heal and reconnect. Creating the space you call home brings with it so much comfort because, mostly, even with those close to us, many do not understand because they may never have experienced what you have or even comprehend what you have.

Forgive yourself and give yourself grace too - Many times when we have lost, we go through a turmoil of emotions that we end up saying a lot. There is a rage that hits, and many don't know they were capable of it. With emotions, we feel very entitled and robbed. Many can be cruel to themselves as they see themselves as failures because they deem this life as one that should be possible in every shame and form. Through it all, forgive yourself for being hard on yourself. Also, forgive yourself for being disgusted with your body. And then give yourself grace and a pat on the shoulder for every mishap and roadblock in life that comes to teach us something. Give yourself grace.

Process the event - After everything calms down, process the event so that you can empty yourself. Cry, feel it all, question God or whichever high spirit you pray to, feel the disappointments and reminisce. Grieve so that you can create space within yourself to continue. The cloud will set off one day, but take each day as it comes. Be with people who allow you to feel things without judgment. Don't be made to feel that it is time to get over things because nobody gets anything. You simply learn to navigate your life around that void and live with it for all eternity.

Binding - Birth of any gestation age leaves a void in your womb. It does not have to be overrated and expensive. Any wrap you have or a long scarf that you have in the house would be fine. There is also not one way of doing this. You want to wrap your belly from the hips up to your rib cage. The one thing that can help you feel closed in and 'held' is binding. Binding your belly can provide a lot of physical comforts. It provides warmth, too. There really is no one way fits all where binding is concerned. Every country in the world does their binding differently and for different reasons, but the benefits are for the same outcome, to provide core support and emotional support and hold you together.

Keeping warm - This is also vital to your recovery. When you think of how the heat makes you feel, it enhances blood flow and leaves you with a 'feel-good warmth that a cold feeling does not. In Kenya, they say cold travels from the feet up and therefore anyone of childbearing age should cover up from the bottom up. The chest area would always be covered up when you are breastfeeding because there is the belief that with birth you become so open that you are open to everything, like infections and the colds. Back home reason one would be covered up even in the heat is it is very easy for cold to set in. When you are breastfeeding, the chest being exposed to cold affects milk production.

The reason we wear '**dera**' is that the seam on the sides of the arms can be opened enough to pass the breast for feeding without exposing the chest area. Deras are free dresses made of really soft cotton that we wear a lot in Kenya for various occasions. Their print is vibrant and colorful, and it is usually accompanied by what we call a '**leso**' or **kanga.**

Allowing your body to rest - When one rests, clarity comes to become. When your mind is racing, you remain in a mode that is tiring for your body, both physically and emotionally as well. Rest calms you and your body so that you can progress. With every opportunity, allow yourself to just be without thought because your body will thank you for it. Maybe not immediately, but it will in the long run.

Eating nourishing warm food - In any phase of recovery, back in Kenya, they do not support consuming cold food. Warm food has a way of filling you up and how it leaves you feeling. The contentment that you feel after eating warm meals is incomparable. The meals have to be nourishing to assist in your energy and mental wellness. If it is not warm, it can be at room temperature but never cold.

> *Therapy is not only for the broken. Naomie Karemi KAINGU*

Acknowledge your feelings - You will be hurt for a while. The 'cloud' will set in, but know where it is enough and where to allow yourself to be. Sometimes people mean well, they simply do not know how to say things. If something that was said triggers you remove yourself from the place or say something calmly if you can. There will be days you feel ok to get up and do stuff, and other times you will be triggered by something you see. Allow yourself to feel the feelings without scrutinizing yourself. Don't act or 'feel' normal when you are not. Acknowledge that you are hurting and allow yourself to find peace and calm through it.

Talk to someone - Many people will tell you that many times when they have spoken with others and not the person they lay with, it brought a feeling of release. Sometimes you need to speak to someone else who is not attached to you emotionally to understand and realize a point of action. I like to normalize speaking to therapists because therapy is not only for the broken. Therapists help to ensure you are looked after and supported after the support network goes back to live their lives. Therapists step in when families can no longer support them.

Steaming/body works - You could treat yourself to vaginal steaming too. This would feel like you are giving yourself a vaginal spa moment. The heat that penetrates from down below is known for not only bringing in the comfortable and earthen but it speeds up your recovery. It helps to expel any leftover blood that would normally be stuck on the wall of your womb and inside your body to loosen and come out. Many women in the postpartum period even experience bleeding much more, but for a shorter period. Bodywork is basically 'touch'. Touch has many healing benefits. When someone touches you intentionally with a massage or cuddle, you feel safe and supported. Many people break down because of what touch means to them and if they needed to be held at that moment. Touch encourages people to feel and be vulnerable.

Add warming herbs and spices to your meals and drinks - In Kenya we love our Chai. Chai is made of some very delicious spices and there are many others that you can use, including ginger, cinnamon, turmeric, cardamom, etc. There are many recipes you can find online for many drinks that you can create yourself without having to buy so much extra.

What I love about spices and herbs is many homes already have something that can be used. I will share a Chai recipe at the end of this chapter for you to try :-). There is also a sweet banana recipe that we cook for our postpartum and anyone recovering because sweet is always welcomed. The recipe includes spices like cardamom and coconut cream, making it so wholesome and warming too.

Another thing you need to know is how to use herbs. Not all herbs work the same. Some are potent and some are not. But I remember my grandmother saying to me she would pluck them intentionally whilst communicating with the plant, almost having a conversation on what she needed that plant and what she was going to use it for. She always said; Quill your herbs before using them. Let them sit before using the herbs so that they become thaw and weak. This way, the strength of the medicine in the herb will not be too much for your body. Be mindful when you are using herbs for their strength value. If you are using the herb for tincture, boiled it as is because one needs the strength as high as possible to combat what it needs to.

Take things slowly. Don't rush into being normal and everything back to how it was. Sometimes between your ears, you may feel that you can until you get up and realize you are not ready still. Allow yourself to just be and build 'normalcy', slowly adding tasks or duties as you see fit. If you feel like resting, allow yourself to. If you feel like staying away from it all, which is very normal, let yourself be.

Create a moment to speak with one another calmly. This one can be hard and one to do gently. Even for myself, who has been together with my husband for over a decade, sometimes having a meaningful conversation without feeling attacked is difficult. It is so much easier to type to each other 'I love you xxxxxx than to address how you feel. And especially after an event or incident, emotions are still rife and can remain like that for a while. It is normal to feel triggered and if this is how both of you feel, consider involving outside help like a mediator or a counselor to allow you both to speak your truths without getting emotional and ending up saying things you might live to regret.

Give thanks - this one is big and has been encouraged a lot ancestrally. I remember my mother reminding me to always give thanks to my womb for carrying the life that I lost, even if for a month. To always remember what my birth gave me, a baby that did not stay, teaching in life (maybe I would never have known how to hold space without growing into this calling and experiencing myself what support in these moments can do to someone).

Journaling - I love this one the most. For me personally, journaling is like speaking to a therapist who is not present, who will not make me feel judged, and who allows me to put down exactly how I feel. The other thing why I love journaling is the fact that later on, you could read the same words back to yourself exactly how you wrote them. No Chinese messenger where a sentence will be deleted, 2 added and the whole end message changes from the original. With this, you can see your progress and appreciate the journey you have traveled through because it will affirm to you what a strong person you really are and enhance the traits you never even knew you had to start with!

You could journal together with your partner if they are interested. Many times they would try to support you, hurting in disguise. It may be a moment where they would flip or react irrationally, but many partners take the role of the 'captain' to keep everything going, including supporting you, and put themselves on the back burner. Whilst they can do that and get away with it for a while, It may backfire. Allowing them to note down how they feel would give you an understanding without arguments or feeling some kind of way. When both of you are emotionally hurt, not much conversation would happen.

Don't lose yourselves through the process - Through the process of grieving, it is very easy to want to shut down and remain in a hole of your own with no one around you. Whilst that may be comforting for a while, it is not healthy. Allow others to check and love on you also as you process and heal.

Choose your battles - Where family is concerned, if people offer to support you through the postpartum period, regardless of how your relationship has been, the news of a newborn baby has nothing to do with it. Ancestrally people did not gather around because they all loved you but because they understood the meaning of community and it has been the ways of our people. Do not refuse help off of a proud moment and regret it later on. Mostly, those who step in to offer support heal their experiences from your experience. Allow them to see and acknowledge the importance of what support can do. Maybe they did not experience it themselves. By allowing them to support you, they may learn to pay it forward even more

WHY IS THE LESO (KANGA) SACRED IN EAST AFRICA?

In many indigenous cultures, there was and still is a piece of cloth that has sustained a lot of RITES. In Congo, for example, they have the Chitenge which we call 'kitenge' in Kenya. Kitenge is a cloth that can be measured according to its need. It can be used to make dresses and clothes of every style and every kind. The kanga is one that is very East African, actually.

> *Many claim it these days, but it IS East African. Naomie Karemi KAINGU*

In Kenya, when a daughter is born, they are blessed with a Kanga by their maternal grandmothers. This becomes a piece of material or cloth that she will use as she grows. Many women would have a piece in their handbags or bags everywhere they went because we say kanga is **'stiri'** meaning 'to conceal or dignity'. Especially in the childbearing years when many do not have regular menstruation cycles, you never know when a Kanga might come to rescue as the prints are so beautiful they become a fashion accessory so fast.

The beauty of the Kanga is that it can be very personalized with the print, colors, texture, and message that is printed at the bottom. Usually, people would choose the printed message according to who they are gifting the Kanga. If it is for your mother-in-law, for example, the message would reflect that with respect, love, and gratitude. If it is for a wedding, messages would usually be along the line of congratulations, prayers, well wishes, etc. For the baby's 40-day celebration, it is the same, in lines of prayers for good health, prosperity, etc. So when you got one as a gift, it is always a souvenir that has many treasures. And because it is personalized, it will never be the same as what you would find in the market and therefore makes for a special gift.

The uses of the Kanga are vast. When not cut into two and the pieces are still attached, the length of it is long enough to use for providing strength when the pelvic pain sets in. It can be used to pull on strength for the laboring person when upright. In its full length, it can also be used for massaging the body in the Kenyan way of pregnancy and postpartum, which is very different. When cut into two pieces, we use it to wrap the parts of the body individually. It can be used to carry babies/children, to carry loads, or to wrap baskets to carry along. It can be used as a bedsheet to wrap a newborn baby, as a receiving cloth for newborn babies, etc.

As you prepare to try again, know that the next pregnancies after losing a baby are difficult. They come with a lot of fear, anxiety, and guilt. There are ways you can help yourself go through the months step by step and celebrate the milestone still. It may be hard and those around you also need to realize that having another baby will not replace the one you lost.

How to Handle the Anxiety, Fear, and Stress that Come with Pregnancy After Loss? Focus on one day at a time. Easier said than done, right? Pregnancies after losing a baby can make every trimester triggering. Pay attention to what is going well each day and how you are feeling. Pay attention also to the progress of the baby recognizing and connecting with the kicks when they become recognizable. Remember your scans and how the baby was moving and is healthy. Remember, each pregnancy is different, and that you miscarried, had an infant loss, or had a stillbirth does not mean this pregnancy will end that way. Put positive energy through mediating and connecting as a family.

Your emotions through the next journey will have many highs and lows. Some highs will be very high and the lows the lowest too. It may be something you can pin down and sometimes just your 'human' you dealing with things. Don't always expect to be happy and joyful all the time - We all have good and bad days when we are not pregnant, so don't expect it to be joyful and happy all the time. Remind yourself that being pregnant again can be a scary experience.

Journal - Writing your feelings is the most healing way you can imagine. By emptying yourself of everything not directly to anyone but putting down in your own words, your rawness and brokenness can heal you throughout your pregnancy after loss. Your feelings of grief will still be there and having a personal journal to vent in will help you process those feelings of grief and the new feelings of being pregnant. It is the hardest thing to do, to accept the void and celebrate the now. Journaling has many benefits, including it will show you in time your progress and the journey you have both traveled

Celebrate Milestones - Celebrating does not mean you dismiss that there was a baby who did not stay in your family. By celebrating milestones, you get to be grateful for the steps you are taking, evolving, and growing. Many women say that their anxiety and stress diminish when they get past the date of their loss. Celebrating those milestones in pregnancy helps you focus on the next goal. These weeks are critical in pregnancy whether it is going from one trimester to another, viability (24 weeks), lung development (32 weeks), and full-term at 39 weeks helps you look forward to what is coming by ticking your progress.

Take Care of Yourself - Life starts with your health being ok. If you intend to grow, nurture, and birth a baby, your general health is important in how your pregnancy will come to be. It is not a guarantee that by being healthy your baby will stay, but every decision that you needed to make if made beforehand helps in achieving this. Do what you need to do to make this the most healthy pregnancy. Celebrate your milestones by scheduling yourself a prenatal massage and let them know you have a stressful pregnancy and need to relax.

Seek a Therapist, Coach, or Grief Counselor - Speaking to professionals can help you combat and deal with things positively. Sometimes it may just be an affirmation from someone to guide you in the right direction. And many times you will not find that in your own home. It helps seek help outside so that you can function inside. Do not go through this pregnancy alone without talking to someone if you have constant feelings of anxiety, fear, and stress. These feelings are common, but if you want extra support, seek a therapist who can support you and provide you with some coping skills to make this pregnancy as calm as possible.

> *Remember that your story matters and when you share it, and with whom you share it, it is ok to do so. - Naomie Karemi KAINGU*

Remember that just because nobody knew about your pregnancy or saw your bump grow (if it did) does not mean that your pregnancy does not matter. Do not expect linear progress as you recover. It is very normal to feel you are moving two steps forward and 4 steps back sometimes through the process. Expectations in grief are inevitable. Some people, even those in our midst, will expect you to be xyz by xyz time. Let them realize that in this pace, you follow your own pace and allow for flow.

Create two lists to work through this process. The first list will be for the people who lift you up in prayer, physical support, and hold space without leaving you feeling judged. The people who did not make it on this list didn't make it in for a reason. Be mindful of the energy they bring and if it is not serving you, stay clear of it. The second list should be of everything that is bringing you joy, calm, tranquillity, and comfort.

This one is a list to hand over to your husband/boyfriend/partner

Thirteen

CELEBRATE YOUR PROGRESS

… every single one of them, no matter how small. The postpartum period can be brutal because a lot of things remain repetitive, especially in the first few months. Sometimes it is hard to keep up with the pace and see the journey you may have traveled to. The children grow right under your nose. You hardly see the difference because you are with them throughout.

In Kenya, we say **'shukuru Mungu uzidi kubarikiwa'** (*Shu-ku-ru *Mu-ngu- *U-zi-di *Ku-ba-ri-ki-wa*) means one should give thanks and show gratitude so that they can continue receiving. With grace comes multiple.

Normalize praising yourself for the hard work done. Normalize praising each other for the small wins achieved. And remember every pregnant person and every pregnancy has its own normal. Not all pregnancies are miserable and exhausting.

As new parents - Trust your guts until proven otherwise. Parenting will challenge you both as parents and test you on all levels you can not fathom. Discussing how you want to raise your child/children beforehand will avoid certain discussions being discussed later on in the journey of parenting. Agreeing with each other as parents make correcting and deciding on what is right for your family easier. Be open about certain topics if they trigger incidents or events in your own childhood and maybe involve your elders to chime in to help you make sense of certain decisions.

I can tell you from experience that parenting is isolating and can be very lonely sometimes. Finding a group of others can help, but everyone will most likely be going through the same things as you. It helps when you can share notes, the triumphs, and the tribulations with others who *get it*, but be aware that being alone and being comfortable, especially in this neck of the woods in the first world countries, is the norm. These days there are many support groups online that you could join which can be helpful.

The postpartum is also about thriving - Not only surviving. Don't fall for the narrative that postpartum is only about misery and hardships. In the Western world, Pregnancy, Birth, and postpartum is an industry that is growing more than rapidly with tones of appropriation and revamping of other people's cultures. And therefore, it is very clear that the narrative of struggle and looking for fixes benefits someone. Products that could almost open a home pharmacy are flung left, right and center, and instead of people seeking knowledge from within, you find many first-time parents jumping at every 'solution' proposed out there because suddenly it is not normal for a newborn baby to cry and guaranteed there is a bottle of fix that can help them.

They cry - babies, especially newborns cry. It might drive you crazy sometimes, but whatever you do, do not take any of it personally. No baby cries for no good reason even though sometimes they will drop lines like 'they need to clear their lungs', babies cry as their way of communicating with you. In time, you will learn what makes them cry a certain way, but as they only arrived home, be gentle and available for your baby. You are the only person who can comfort them. Do not despair or feel inadequate.

Overwhelming - It can get cumbersome and overwhelming because babies need you 210% and constantly too. It will feel you are doing the same time repetitively, but go with the pace and don't think you can do extra xyz, otherwise you will run yourself to the ground.

Let go - you cannot hold on to power in this mode. Your boss is the one in your arms and their needs are vast in the beginning. Let go of the 'perfect syndrome. Be extra mindful of your own mental well-being. You might sometimes find something so small triggers you or sends you into emotional turmoil. Sobbing from pregnancy (with some people) and right into postpartum is very normal, especially in the beginning from the accumulation of exhaustion, overwhelming doubt, etc. Sometimes a certain voice will come and ruin your peace with doubt and sadness in the beginning. It is normal, but know what triggers you and how to distract yourself from it, too.

> *It is always easy to see others doing better than yourself. Trust me, everyone goes through struggles in the beginning. Naomie Karemi KAINGU.*

Comparison - this one is a killer if nothing else. Instagram parenting can make you look inadequate and incapable. Many look in control and well done. They couldn't possibly be struggling or going through the same struggles as you. Everyone goes through the same struggles in the beginning, even if they have given birth before because every pregnancy and baby is different. They went through similar experiences to get o where you are seeing them. Your turn will come. Be patient with yourself.

Parenting is lonely and can be isolating, too. If you have other children, consider involving them with all the age-appropriate stuff that they can help you with. Remember, everyone within the family goes through the void, even pets, and they need to learn what their places are and what the coming of this new baby means to them. Being involved in mother-baby groups will in some ways enable you to see that actually, your own struggles are not too huge. Changing space and energy too can be beneficial. Go with the notion that 'distance makes the heart grow fonder' and be absent from home for a significant amount of time with other parents and their babies just to recharge your energy.

Gratitude/Grace - Through the whole recovery process and developing as parents, remember to give yourself grace. Parenting is a journey that many signs out of because they realize later on that it is not meant for them. So loving this little person for 18 years to start with and for all eternity will come with a lot of prices and sacrifices. Many people clock out and if you can stand through and through and tall, give yourself grace. By doing so, and celebrating all your wins no matter how small, maybe finally, your child hits the milestone after seeing all others do it earlier in your mama group or family, rejoice. Reaching milestones is not a given to anyone. Every child will develop at their own pace, even when you bore all of them, they will all reach their potential in their time.

Do not compare your children either and live in misery because now they should have been doing xyz, and the sister did it much earlier.

Do not mourn for a future you have not lived in yet. Allow it to show itself. There will be many transitions that will be scary for a parent. Many times you are not sure if you, as a parent, are capable even, but remember that the challenges come to prepare you for greatness. They come to challenge you to think outside of your comfort zone. They come to allow us to change our ways and swerve us in the directions we never thought we could look at.

Children do not come with manuals. Allow yourself to make mistakes as you both explore and learn the ways around each other. When a baby is born into a family, everyone within that home needs to adjust themselves, including you. You have never been a parent before, nor were you ever a parent with x amount of children. So come to terms with that fact, embrace it and then own it. Back in my native country, Kenya, the older children are involved with the upbringing of a sibling. This way, they build the connection from a tender age. Young girls are taught how to carry their siblings on their backs from a tiny age so that their parents can work.

The community and family have always been in alignment with each other and their needs are met within the 'unit'. Older children go through feelings of displacement and everyone needs to adjust to that so that there is no feeling of too much time being taken away or attention being lost because now there is a new baby. This can in the long term create spite among siblings. Some may show their anxiety through emotions with tears and feeling abandoned. Remember to involve them in normal decision-making (age-appropriate) so that they may feel like part of the family through the change. For many, the coming of a newborn baby brings with it a lot of fear, anxiety, anger, jealousy, abandonment, and feeling displaced.

There are many ways you can empty your 'being' and relieve yourself. One is by journaling. Putting things down yourself helps in so many ways. You do not end up lumbering your partner with extra worries because they are probably going through their own adjusting, it enables you to fill your lungs to continue breathing. Putting things down in your own words enables you to read them back to yourself later on and see the progress you have really made. The beauty of putting things down is also the fact that one day, when you can sit and look back at the events, you will read the words back to you as you felt back in the day. Nothing altered, nothing corrected, your exact words which can bring closure and healing.

> *Parenting is like birth. It demands a level of holding on and letting go, too. Naomie Karemi KAINGU.*

The invisible load - Is real. Many times, your thoughts don't just stop with you thinking about your baby and when the next feed will be. You attempt to bring the pieces together in your head. Many times you try to make sense of things that just happened or how you remember the birth to have been. You manage the other children (if any) at the same time that you recover. But because parenting is not applaudable, nobody will knock on your door and clap for you for the 90th diaper you have changed... the load remains simply that; invisible.

Parenting, though we function through it, is hard. For many around us, it is very hard for them to see because we keep things rolling. As parents, we normalize it all and many times show up even when we are broken because parenting demands we do. No one will clap for the number of diapers you have changed. Nobody will pat you on your back for sticking through it, even with very little sleep. Nobody will applaud you for juggling it throughout sometimes, even when you didn't feel you could. So do not let anyone tell you how to parent, how to do whatever, and when to do it either.

Remember, everything you did to arrive at your last destination and applaud yourself for sticking through it, for continuing, even though sometimes it felt like the entire world was judging you and scrutinizing you. It can be hard to give yourself credit even if you remember the journey and all its hurdles.

> **CHECK-IN WITH YOURSELF**: *'Hello, how have you been since we last saw each other? Naomie Karemi KAINGU.*

Once in a while, it is very healthy to check in with yourself. Catch up with who you were and who you have become as well. As a mother and as a father, it is ok for you to stop and catch your own breath. Having a baby does not mean you stop chasing your dreams and aspirations. Being a parent does not mean your whole life revolves around your child either. Being parents, your children will always be extra of your relationship. The focus starts and ends with you.

It is very important to keep track of your own progress throughout the journey of parenting. Growth is both ways. Just as you are eager to watch your baby grow, hit the important milestones, develop well and become their own selves, it is important not to forget yourself. Parenting does not mean you leave everything behind, your dreams, your aspirations, and your wants. Parenting demands you also grow so that they can reflect on your journey, too. Do not be too comfortable with them now because they will leave the nest one day. They will become their own people, and they will leave you so that they can do the things they were ordained to do through you.

Grow with them. Grow together so that you can uplift each other too.

> *Children come through you, not from you. They are here for a purpose. Don't quit or forget yourself. Naomie Karemi KAINGU.*

You cannot level up to society and its expectations of parenthood: Society has put so much weight on the shoulders of women and parents alike from the moment they test positive. A journey that should start calmly and be one that brings joy and togetherness, is often looked at or frowned upon as something that is almost a bother to folk who will not carry the pregnancy, birth the baby or raise them up. After having children, you realize that in the eyes of society, mothers can't:

1. **Complain** (because who told you to have children?) - Parenting is work. There are people who decide to take the leap of parenting wholeheartedly, but that does not mean that it is peaches and candies all the time. It is hard work, one that is rewarding when you see the work you put in sometimes and other times. It can simply become suffocating.
2. **Cry** (why are you crying? Did you think it was easy when you were wishing for them?) - Emotions are part of this journey and anybody that says otherwise has not raised another human being, especially a child. There will be times you can not do much but cry it out. Crying helps relieve the heart and allows you to breathe in those moments when you have everything right by the child and nothing seems to work.
3. **Get tired** - of what? (you do nothing!) - Nobody is going to clap for the 96 diapers you change throughout the day. Nobody will see in figures, the things you will do as a parent so they do not expect that you would get tired even. Tiredness does not equate to physical tiredness only. There are parents raising children with medical needs that the list of things that mentally need to be arranged and followed up on is exhausting. Silently worrying if your child is hitting the milestones, growing well, happy and functioning like they should do is exhausting. Tiredness cannot be measured. If you are tired, take time out. You need to function around your children and family to raise them.

4. **Sleep** (You're lazy!)–When you think of the number of times you probably got up in the night to attend to the needs of your child, why then is it a crime to sleep in the day when you can so that you can continue?
5. **Rest** (you'll have plenty of time for that after they grow up) - When they are still young, rest is your best friend. Think of the routines and how they occur in the day. If you have a child that sleeps during the day, you see that before they go down to sleep, they can be extremely hyper. Over-tiredness, cranky, weepy. Once they sleep, their mood changes and their energy ups too. Parenting demands you can match up to the needs of your child from the moment they are up again. Do not dismiss the part where rest is vital in how you would parent because it can get overwhelming quickly. A parent who is not rested is more prone to reacting abruptly and causing harm than one who is. REST UP!
6. **Get pregnant again** (are you crazy? How many more kids do you need?) - How many children one has should be nobody else's business. When you stop at only one child, you will be lumbered with. " When is the next one coming? They need a sibling.. so the number of children you decide to have should be your choice and nobody else's. "
7. **Quit work** (how will you support your child?)–Your mental health is important. Unfortunately, there are situations that come up at places of work that demand that one chooses between their growth, happiness or mental health. If it does not work, there are many other doors to try
8. **Work** (who will take care of the child?)—As parents, we are our children's mirrors. They watch and see what we do and will inevitably copy. As parents, we want to show them to be someone in a society of any rank. You need to work. By working, you will provide for them and they would learn that things don't fall from the sky, you have to work for them.

9. **Leave them at the nursery** (Don't let others raise them!!) - As much as we love them to bits, sometimes we need to leave them in the care of other people so that we can function elsewhere. It enables them to be adaptable and learn things they may not learn from only you. There will come a time when they will need more than their mama or their father.
10. **Be a stay-at-home parent** (The Poor husband, who works too hard and his wife stays at home!!)–Another one that is not up to society to detect how you live or what you become. If as a couple you have decided that it is better for one of you to stay at home and raise the children, good for you! There are children who do not thrive in daycares or in the care of others for various reasons. Daycares as we know them are a breeding ground for sickness and some children, cannot thrive in such environments where the sickness lingers for so long and by the time they are recovering, the round comes back to them again, not allowing them time to recover.
11. **Be single** (nobody wants a woman with kids) - Depending on what the situation was, nobody becomes single willingly. Given there are some people who choose to for various reasons, but then again, it took two to create those babies. In Swahili we have a saying '***ukitaka mgomba upende na ndizi zake!*** which translates to when you love the banana tree, love it with its fruits.
12. **Go out for fun** (why are you leaving your children to have fun?) - don't forget you. Learning the ropes and finding your way around parenting is very normal, but don't stay there. Reconnect with the world again.

So, as you can see from the list, you will never match up to other people's expectations of you. Be the best you can be, knowing you are doing right by your children and family. The notion that, once you become a mother/parent, your life must revolve around the children, and all your ambitions, aspirations, wants, and needs must be packed up and locked away is suffocating. You grow together with your children. They watch you grow. Be an example they will always look upon and hope they want to be like their mother/father.

Sadly, 90% of these phrases are spoken by other women, which is very sad to hear. If only we would go back to Ancestral wisdom, where Birth was celebrated as an event that brings people together and renews the lineage, we would understand what new parents need in their moment of 'becoming' is love, support, and understanding. Where raising children is a joint effort among loved ones and the community at large.

Women have various events in their lives. There are those strictly on anti-conception where the anti-conception method failed, and a child is still conceived. There are cases of women raped who conceive. Birth is life and life should be celebrated regardless of how it was conceived

Fourteen

THRIVE...DON'T SURVIVE

Thriving may seem like a far-fetched achievement in the immediate postpartum period because the postpartum period can be brutal, to begin with. Please be gentle with yourself and stay in the moment. Don't rush to get out of it because this is the moment of evolution for you as the birthing person and also for your family. Slow the pace by accepting where you are at and taking things as they come to you.

When you feel like you have all balls in the air, your whole body aches, your mind is still in overdrive, your hormones are all over the place, you are wearing the biggest incontinence pads you ever set your eyes on; you are bleeding and probably still cramping, your breasts are too full, or you are worried you don't have enough milk for your little one; the list can be endless, and your mental load can get overwhelming too fast.

Your biggest support and sanity here is rest. Take things slowly, do not rush. Between your ears, you will feel ready to take on the world. There is a reason ancestrally birthing people remained away from the outside world and energy to recuperate and recover first before being reintroduced back into their clans and communities. As a newborn person, you are still very open spiritually, emotionally, and physically. You are more tearful than you normally are pre-pregnant.

You are more receptive energy-wise, which can be harmful, especially if the energy disrupts your routine and how your family structure is set up. An example would be when someone walks in and suggests something that you agree to so fast because you find yourself in the 'save-me mode' and what you hear makes sense when in fact it is not how you have always lived your lives as a family.

The placenta is said to be the size of a dinner plate. When you think the whole organ detached from your womb after childbirth, you will then understand the need for you to take things slowly and slow your pace, too. Anybody who knows you have had a baby should expect you to slow down, too. Even in your home after childbirth, you are NOT the host. Everyone should come and hold you and celebrate with you and nurture you. Don't bring haste in this sacred phase of your life before it is time, because it will not be very gentle with you. Later on, it will hit you like a boomerang.

A time will come when you will sprint into action again or be up and down like you wish to, but not at this moment in your postpartum period.

If you have family or a community behind you willing to avail themselves for you, accept the support even if only for some small things like playdates for your other children, meals delivered to you either through a set-up meal train where people pick a day they would avail themselves to do something for your family. Use your energy for duties nobody else can do, like loving and nurturing your newborn baby and bringing your family into the circle of change. Allow others to be a part of your journey differently, doing the rest of the things for you and your family.

In the Netherlands, where a maternity nurse comes to your home for the first 8 or 10 days after childbirth, it can be a relief to know you have someone at hand for you, six hours in the day. My tip for you at this moment, in your quiet moment, write all your questions down to ask the following day. Ask her to confirm things with you whilst you still have her coming because she is the intermediary between the hospital and the midwife.

At this moment, it can feel like you have your hands in all pies at the same, especially if there are other children at home that need attention too. Don't be disheartened, though, the immediate postpartum period is not to be undermined. It is a moment for everyone to adjust and evolve together. This is a moment of doubt, grieving, and tests, but also confirmation of your ability to function as a parent. Take each day as it comes.

You cannot do more than that.

In your postpartum period, it can be difficult to know how to delegate duties and responsibilities. It also depends highly on why are in your circle and available to support you. Support usually comes from those who see your need to be supported and offer it wholeheartedly, without expectations or hold it as a debt. In all honesty, nobody will clap for all the 97 diapers you have been changing. The tasks assigned to us as parents will not always be recognized. ***Don't wait for recognition. You will hurt and lose yourself***. There is no medal for the perfect pregnancy, the perfect birth, or the perfect parent.

Parenthood is beautiful, but it is also work and hard work too. So act like you are going to work every day once the difficult days have passed (usually the first 3/4 days). Take it as a calling and be realistic about it, too. If you got out of bed and went to work with a hungry stomach, you would not function. Your mental capacity will be decapitated, your concentration ability will be affected.. how then do you propose or even think it is possible to take care of a baby with an empty stomach?

How would you do that?

1. Let go of perfectionism–It is a scam where parenting is concerned
2. Choose your battles wisely. Sometimes you will find it's not worth winning an argument or situation. Sometimes none of it makes sense
3. Stop trying to do it all, you will risk running yourself to the ground
4. Normalize having a normal routine every day. Shower, look presentable, and feel good
5. Take it slow, a time to do the running around will come
6. Enjoy the moment to sit and feed your baby. It won't be like that always
7. Delegate chores and duties so you are not snowed down
8. Ask for help without feeling like a failure. It is better to ask than struggle behind closed doors
9. Don't feel a certain way about sitting or lying down. Your body is using a lot of energy to keep you and the baby healthy
10. Dishes will always be there. Let them be for a moment while you breathe
11. Accept that other people's support is meant well. This one has many first-time parents wanting to prove to the world they have it together
12. Let things slide. In this phase of parenting, you are very open and receptive, sieve information that is useful, and let the rest be

THE FIRST TEACHER

.. Ever, Is the parent and we are our children's mirrors too. How we speak to our children, they learn and project it to others, too. Binding in the early moments was encouraged by keeping everyone else away so that your focus was on your newborn baby and your family. Use the time to speak to them and let them learn your voice. Speak greatness to your child and help them see the world through your eyes. Talk about your own family history or lineage with them to enable them to react in their own way.

Babies grasp and understand more than we give them credit for. Back home in Kenya, babies are even allowed to mingle with other babies of different ages to grasp what they can in order to develop themselves. Them being told the family stories was part of the upbringing. Names were mentioned of family members that were still present and those who had gone before them too so that the family lineage was understood from an early age.

Bonding happens with speech contact, therefore make it your mission to connect with your baby through talk, touch, play and embrace. Don't stop in their baby's times, keep the connection through these aspects as they grow up. You will be surprised how much of the information you shared with them as children they would remember later on.

Fifteen

IMPERFECTLY PERFECT

Imperfectly *perfect* is what parenting is naturally.

Allow yourselves to make mistakes. From the start, allow yourself to take on parenting with flaws. Don't Perfect anything because life in generation is a journey into discovery and teachings. Parenting is similar. Allow things to take their course.

Allow yourself to feel, to experience, and learn from the whole discovery and journey because it is a journey of discovery. There will be many trials and tribulations but also triumphs through the journey of parenting and therefore being able to look back and tap on your backs for accomplishing those milestones should be amongst the things you do when you sit and track back on where you are based on where you started.

No one is born knowing how to parent. With knowledge, trials, and mistakes, you web in the art of parenting and being a child, too. You learn from each other and are entwined as a family unit; you evolve together. Parenting is a skill we learn over time, and it is never a one-moment timing either. There are no expiration dates, you simply evolve together. It is a task granted to us that evolves with time. Allow yourself to grow through it.

It evolves with time because growth comes in phases. Every phase is a milestone for both the parents and the children. For the children, there is reaching and achieving the milestones. For the parents, there is the doubt of not knowing if they are equipped for the task as parents and then seeing how it all 'pears up'. It demands a lot of holding on so that you as parents can instill virtues that will enable your baby to be a citizen of the nation that is respectful, hardworking, honest, etc. It demands a lot of holding on to allowing one to make mistakes because the children did not come with manuals to start with.

> *Parenting after the birth of your baby will be one of life's events that will test you to your core - Naomie Karemi KAINGU.*

Parenting comes in many variations, don't take each other for granted. Whilst each one is making sense of things and trying to stay in their own bubble, don't forget to check in with each other. In parenting, there is no competition, nor is there the 'bad guy', as we like to call it. Whatever you decide should stem from both of you as parents for the better of yourselves.

Don't keep the focus on only holding the family together, but strive to instill resilience in each other. There will be times when one will feel strongly about something. That is the moment for the 'other' parent to listen out and try to understand why that is. When one feels low, the one feeling great will hold the space. You will not both be deflated. Don't allow it to happen.

Don't keep your focus on finding out where the other one is at and finding solutions. Only hold each other, but allow each other to be held too. Trust comes from allowing each other to feel vulnerable around each other and trusting each other's support and intentions.

Let gratitude be the foundation you set up on your journey of parenting. Understand that because they did not come with manuals, what you are doing at the moment and time is the best decision. Of course, you will have moments where you will doubt your decisions and if you thought about them rationally, but you can always learn and be better than people and as parents.

Be mindful as parents because we are our children's mirrors. Watch how you speak with one another in front of them or their eras reach. Parenting can remind us of our own childhood and the worst moments of that, too. Be aware of a couple of your own triggers. When you parent, sometimes your own experiences can resurface whether you acknowledged or honor that. Learning about your triggers can help you evaluate what your child may go through at that moment and time.

Triggers that take you back to the dark places in your own experience are worth speaking with professionals about. You can mention to your midwife what emotions or feelings you are struggling with and see if together you can find a solution.

Feeling overwhelmed as a newborn parent is very normal. Be mindful of how long you feel a certain way because it should not remain like it for a long time. Be cautious, what you do with the emotions matter

Remember, hurt people can heal. Naomie Karemi KAINGU.

Sixteen

YOUR OTHER/OLDER CHILDREN

Having a baby brings so much anxiety within the family home. Everyone needs to adjust to the new family member and understand what their presence means and their positions within the home. This is so true for older siblings. It can be daunting to comprehend the change of events for small children. First, they have to understand that the baby that was in your stomach/womb has been born and they are in your home to stay. It might take a while before they comprehend the baby is not being picked by anyone or that the guests that visit did not forget the baby. It's a whole puzzle that needs to sink in slowly.

When you have a second child, please do not forget your first one. Their needs remain the same if not more triggered, because they suddenly must wait or share you with another child. Mostly, you will notice the imbalance with frequent tantrums, fighting for attention, feeling threatened, and probably, more than before, seeking attention.

They too need to adjust to the change, and it is mega for them, too.

It is a known fact that when a sibling is born, the older children recline in age. If they were advanced in certain things, they go back in time. For example, a 4-year-old who was already dry in the night may begin to wet their bed again or try to talk in baby talk to get your attention or to help them remain in the 'needy' phase with you. These moments can also be isolating and maybe threatening because everyone comes with excitement because of the birth, so inevitably for the baby. It is easy for your older children to feel some type of way because their sibling has been born and your focus and attention goes to the new baby instead of them. In these current times, you can involve them in a lot of ways.

If you plan to have them present for the birth of their sibling and speak to them about what they can expect to see, you will be in discomfort, and it is not the baby's fault for example so they are not already putting blame and creating animosity. You could already talk about the stages of labor and how that would feel for you, so they are assured you will be in pain, but it is part of the process, and they cannot save you even if they wanted to. You could take them with you to your scan appointments and allow them to ask questions to your midwife or gynecologist.

If you plan to give birth at home, involve them with setting up the room where their sibling will be born, let them help you prepare the birthing pool, choose the first outfit, and let them know one of the baby's names if they would have multiple names and keep one name a surprise. Allow them to own a moment within the planning so that they feel included.

FIND A BIT OF CALM AMIDST THE CHAOS

Older children's main frustration is the waiting that needs to happen after the birth of a sibling. Suddenly they need to wait for their turn before they can get your attention for many things.

That on its own can create anger and jealousy. There are ways you could try to plan your day in a way that helps everyone get the same attention, not 100% but better than leaving a child to feel left out because of their sibling and therefore brewing resentment.

Create a family day rhythm that prioritizes the older children whilst the baby is still young. A newborn baby's needs are minimal or manageable in the first months. Take care of the older children first, before you care for the baby. Setting up a routine that leads with the older children enables the newborn baby to fit in with the routine. For example, if the older children are in bed at 7:30 pm, then the little one will learn that at after that time the older siblings are quiet, it must be sleep time, and will hopefully follow suit.

Regarding mealtimes, feed the baby first because then you can calmly focus on the rest without having to double up on your attention and you can deal with the needs of your older children.

HOW CAN YOU HELP THEM ADJUST TO THEIR SIBLING?

Talk to them about the changes that will happen when the baby is born and at home with you all. If they were the only children, then talk to them about the needs of a baby and that there will be times you will not be available immediately. They need your attention, but you will attend to them as soon as possible.

Give them the opportunity to ask questions if they have any Children have a huge imagination naturally and therefore, creating space where they can ask questions for you to answer honestly will help them understand instead of them wandering with their own stories in their heads.

Prepare the house ahead of time so that if they are moving rooms, they can adjust to their new room ahead of time without fury that they were indeed moved to make way for their sibling, which will create more animosity than harmony.

Include a gift for your older children to celebrate their sibling. Something that 'the baby picked for their older siblings. It will help warm the meeting. Don't leave the attention only on the baby. You could also plan ahead of time as a family and have gifts for your older child in a cupboard that they open every day during the visiting week, which normally is the immediate postpartum week.

Make a fuss about the first meeting. Make it a special family occasion without an audience when introducing them to their baby brother or sister. There is no knowing how they would react toward the baby, and having other people around creates more anxiety than calm.

Try to keep them in their usual routine. If they go to daycare, let them continue with the routine they know to avoid disruption and confusion. They have their own friends and routine at nursery or daycare, or maybe your own parents look after them on certain days, keep that routine so that when they are gone, you also catch up on your own strength and bring in routine slowly. Keeping them in their known routines helps them stay in what they already know, which in effect will bring calm to their already busy minds.

Involve them in all the planning, like choosing clothes for the baby. Children love to be involved and ask for opinions about certain things within the home. One certainly is where a newborn sibling is. Asking them what set the baby should wear helps them feel 'older' and included.

Include them in other duties like bathing the baby. They could watch whilst you give the baby a bath, and they could also help with putting soap or drying the baby after the bath.

Acknowledge their feelings. It's inevitable that they would feel a little odd and anxious about a new brother or sister. This is like when a guest comes to visit. You need time to warm up to them and get used to their presence. Remind them they are not alone with the big feelings and that you understand them (if you also had siblings yourself, use your own example because that is close to home for them to understand).

Appoint them with certain chores concerning the baby, like taking the diapers in the outside bin, and sorting out the baby's laundry according to color.

Give them attention and cuddles to reassure them that your love for them will not change because there is another baby because you have enough love to share with them all. Remind them they have not been replaced by their baby brother or sister.

Decide ahead of time who will spend the most time with your older children. Inevitably, it would be your partner or your parents/in-laws to ensure that the attention they were receiving before their sibling does not change so much. As the birthing parent, you would spend a lot of time in bed recovering, and therefore, you cannot join him or her in the games or to the playground. Your partner would be the best person to offer this and bring some sort of equilibrium into the house.

Try not to have expectations on how they would react to meeting their sibling.

There is no telling beforehand what their reaction would be. It may be best to introduce the baby to them from the crib so that you can hold them when they show disappointment or emotional outbursts.

Ask your guests who come to bring something small for your older children too, even if it is a used toy from their own children that they can gift.

Ask them how they feel about having a brother or sister after the birth. You could do that through a relative they get on well with, for example, the grandparents or the nanny/babysitter who they trust.

Create time to spend with only your older children individually to help avoid sibling jealousy and rivalry. Small babies are manageable. In the moments when they sleep, create a moment to spend with your older children within the home, tasks that you can do, read them a book, for example, play a game together that is not strenuous for you

Seventeen

THE SNAP-BACK MENTALITY

> *Back home we say 'akizaliwa mtoto na mama pia amezaliwa'. When a baby is born, so is the mother. Naomie Karemi KAINGU*

That you can 'snap back' Is a lie!!! Please don't let any of this mentality get to you, it will destroy your peace and self-esteem too if you believe any of it. Social media has had a way of creating ideologies that are unreal. The typical Instagram births where most of the babies are born in the water, with candles lit, parents singing hymns, and everyone falling in love immediately set their eyes on each other. As much as social media is great at educating, it can be dangerous in how information shared could be taken literally by some people.

The social media vision of parenting is far from reality. Social media projection of the postpartum period where others are boasting of having run marathons literally days or weeks after childbirth is unreal. The truth is this one; If anything will change you to the core and make you see yourself in a different light, it is childbirth. Not only would pregnancy humble you with all the aches, the ducking walking style, and the changing complexion because of hormones that will bring rash, mood swings, and tiredness, childbirth will simply revamp you.

Many think only about the bump and what else they envisage themselves to do once the baby arrives and life goes back to 'normal, whatever normal is. Well, Birth will change you. Birth will make you grow, it will test you, challenge you, and make you question your abilities and capabilities and why you were even blessed with your child. Sometimes you would feel you are in the constant repetitive mode forever because you will, in the beginning, repeat many things. Be patient with the process, it has to take its cause. There is a feeling that childbirth brings with it.

The '**snap-back**' is a westernized or 'today' mentality. After the birth of a baby, nobody snaps back to their old self, the pre-birth self. I mean, 'when a baby is born, so is the mother'. So you are reborn every time you birth your legacy and family addition. Why or how do you want to go back in time? Instagram will be your killjoy in parenting if you keep up with it because there, nobody shares the journey to the last click of the camera. Just like parenting, how many times do you yell to the children standing in front of the camera 'no, take your hand out of your nose, smile, don't frown so much, stand straight up, don't slouch... The only thing we see on social media is the last click, never the journey. So be mindful of what you go by and what you use as guidance.

Take everything with a pinch of salt because 'just because so and so did it and got away with it, does not mean it is normal. And their normal will never be yours either. Remember to love and focus on what matters in your life. Once you become a parent, you will see things differently. There would be things you would need or choose to pay attention to and those that drain you and make you feel unhappy and unappreciated are the ones to drop. Everyone goes through a change in the childbearing years.

Your focus is loving on yourself because the babies will grow and each one of them will go to and do their own thing. So, through the parenting journey, do not leave yourself behind in the name of love.

Remember to fill your own lungs first before helping others. Sometimes it may mean removing yourself from the situation so that they can all find their own balance. Leave the house, book a babysitter and breathe alone somewhere. When you return, you find that your family would have missed you. Your changing scenery allows for everyone to learn to function without clinging to your ankles like they cannot. It also allows you to free yourself from the constant feeling of being needed because that can be suffocating.

Many women and birthing people alike speak of the struggles years later in a way that reflects the importance of 'being looked after. Many confess to not knowing the importance of letting others nurture them because society in the western world dictates that for you to have gotten it all together, you need to snap back and get on with it even before the clearance at 8 weeks.

This idea of the **strength of the woman is** one of the reasons many cry behind closed doors and why some even have incidents. There is absolutely no medal for being a warrior in giving birth or raising children. As a parent, it is your duty to instill the right virtues in your children and hope that as they grow up, they would put to use what was taught to them. Don't invite comparison into your home because it will rob your peace and the confidence to continue learning and exploring different ways of raising your children. For many parents, the stress of how they 'survived' those first few weeks lingers for years. Don't wait until you cannot recognize yourself in front of the mirror. There will be many versions of yourself you will lose, but talking about your struggle will help you overcome things.

Nobody finds themselves alone - Naomie Karemi KAINGU

Many long to have been 'mothered' because there is something that letting others look after you brings. There is an assurance that settles in when folk come your way to honor, nourish and share in your celebration

- It gives you space to breathe in the presence of others
- It allows you to be vulnerable so that you can grow
- It can boost your self-esteem
- It allows you to find clarity as you are emotionally supported too

Don't listen to that voice - The voice that will tell you sometimes that you are worthless and useless. There will be times when you would look in the mirror and not find yourself. Order that voice aloud and ask it to try you the following day 'not today! Try me tomorrow' because sometimes if you do not call it out it will continue to whisper and remain a secret that is not building you, but breaking you slowly, piece to piece. Let that voice remain useful when you give yourself a pat on your shoulder 'yes! You did goooooood!

Connect with yourself - There is so much solace in being alone. Being alone is not for everyone, but in being alone, you learn to think things through. In being alone, you learn to have a meeting with yourself. Connect or reconnect with yourself. When you arrive back from the hospital, everything will feel different, even now within yourself. There is a new version of YOU that never existed before, and you need to get used to that. There will be duties that you never did before, sounds you didn't hear before, and a feeling of contentment you didn't experience before.

A baby, though small, changes so many things around you, it's unbelievable yet so profound. Through it all, don't lose yourself.

Don't succumb to a level of 'comfort' that will haunt you later on.

You will know when it is time to evolve around this 'duty' because then you will be ready. For now, glue yourself together through the transition. Piece the pieces together as you transition, because this way you will look back and see where you really started and what it indeed was, a journey of growth for you.

Create time for YOU – Self-care is vital so that you can continue to fill into your family. It is not selfish to think about YOU so that your attention and love can come from a place of calm and wholesomeness. You cannot care for or avail yourself to others if you are broken. As parents, we have a tendency of caring for everybody else and forgetting or putting our needs at the back of the radar. *Compassion is not complete if it does not include you. So only be compassionate about everyone around you if you show the same compassion to you first*

Learn to say no - Drop the 'super woman' cape and say no when you cannot take things on. In your process of healing and recovery, you need to let go of other people's expectations that do nothing but add to your workload. If it makes you feel you cannot breathe, it's not one to add to your already overflowing plate. Saying no also does not mean you say no forever, not at that moment, and maybe you will make the request by the following week. Saying no means you are mindful of your own needs. You are prioritizing yourself, and there is nothing wrong with doing that. Live with YOU, because you know YOU better than anyone else. When you take care of YOU first, you would be able to care for others authentically.

Delegate duties - hire that once-a-month cleaner you have been meaning to or wish you could. Get a babysitter so that you can have your free time to do the things that bring you joy. Motherhood or parenthood does not mean your life ends because you have become one. Register for the courses or training you have been wanting to do for a while. You can thrive and be the mother, the parent, the girlfriend, and the wife you imagine yourself to be. Looking after people 24/7 demands a lot from you and believe me, you cannot do that without you being ok first.

In Kenya, we say 'the mood of the house relies on the mother'. If you wake up feeling bad or in a whiney mood, the rest of the family will follow suit. So look after yourself so that you can give the best of yourself to your children. As a parent, your children are a mirror of you

Birth can be one of the most glorious, ecstatic, and empowering experiences of our lives and a potent vehicle for spiritual transformation - if we dare to question everything we have ever been taught.

> Life is not about finding yourself but creating yourself - Naomie Karemi KAINGU

Eighteen

YOUR CARE PROVIDERS

Your care provider could be your midwife, the obstetrician, or the Gynaecologist who will still be in contact with the family after the birth of their baby. In the Netherlands, your midwife takes over your care from the hospital. Maternity nurses support you at home for the first eight days. They are the middlemen between the hospital and the midwife.

The maternity nurses are the intermediary between the midwives and the hospitals and can refer you to where you need to be. That midwives pick up your care when you are sent home from the hospital brings calm and normality within a family unit, especially where you do not need to occupy the hospital bed or be under medical care per se.

Often, they (Care providers) work within protocols and the norm, which means they are stuck with the 6-8 weeks, and the file gets closed. Once I had a student midwife in my evening rooms on the clubhouse app, and the many things we touched on within the room kept saying what I shared that was not in the books! What she meant was that medically they are taught that if the physical outlook looks good, then the birthing person is ok, and the file is then ready to be closed. This knowledge iterates the importance of validating birthing people's experiences because their experience matters. They want to feel that their experiences matter to you, the care provider.

Some birthing people share a completely different story, for example, based on how others made them feel on the day they gave birth. Couples who gave birth vaginally, without medication or interventions, often remember how they received and looked after during the birth of their baby. The negative experiences remain a big part that they share years later.

The norm is that once the suturing (stitches) looks ok, or it's healing, the birthing mother/person is ready. The focus remains on the baby, leaving the well-being of the birthing person or mother somewhat unspoken about at length. Maybe on the day of the appointment, she attempted to look good, clean and put on makeup, then it is concluded she can't possibly be struggling.

ASK HER! How is she doing? Where is she at in her mental load?

Unfortunately, once you can get active physically and sexually, you are ready. By the 8th week, I think many are busy, and this is where the detachment begins. In reality, by that 8th week is when life starts for many families. These are usually the most challenging moments when the support system is almost ending. If people travel down, they are getting ready to leave. This feeling brings a lot of fear and sadness because of **abandonment.**

> *Giving birth is not the most challenging part. The most intricate work is in raising the children. Kenyan saying - Naomie Karemi KAINGU.*

Many newborn mothers/parents cry behind closed doors because of the overwhelm that birth brings. Birth itself comes with a lot of grief, regardless of how it developed. Many things change within her both physically, emotionally, and psychologically. The physiological changes are those that happen to the parents. There would be trauma, swelling, and pain to your perineum, vagina, and anus If they have had a tear during childbirth. Pain depends on many extra factors like if they had an episiotomy (cut) or a natural tear, or a severe tear like a fourth-degree tear that extends as far as into the anal sphincter (the ring of muscle that holds the anus closed).

One can do things to ease the pain, including sitting over a basin with warm water and salt. In my native country, we do not use any concoction of herbs for this. In the hospitals, it is pure salt and warm water. At home, you may find that many would use some Neem boiled to drink and then sit over. They give the Neem internally because Neem has antibiotics factors and is known for combating the fevers that can happen in the immediate postpartum. There is usually a lot of swelling too, and Neem is excellent for that.

If you are in a country where you can access comfrey, lavender, urva Ursi, or shepherds purse, you could try using the mix in a sitz bath which is the same as the classic example of sitting over a basin with warm water, and then this time with this mix. Another way would be to sieve the mixture and have it in a bottle or toilet jug she can use every time she uses the bathroom. Using tissue early postpartum can be very uncomfortable and sensitive for some people.

As a care provider, and from a minority group, I recognize that there is a trust issue for many black families. Healthcare systems have caused harm to minority ethnic groups for the longest time. Many seek support within their communities, sometimes landing on the wrong people while running away from the institution, which is very sad. There have been matches and strikes worldwide where people seek justice in how they are treated compared to other ethnic groups.

The healthcare system has failed minority groups. The rules and protocols within the health care system were written without their involvement or input. Regulations and protocols were written within the care settings, forgetting the minority groups.

Otherwise, there would be an understanding that care is not a one-fits-all and that different minority groups have different needs.

When you have a medic, assume that African people do not need to be helped or taught how to breastfeed a baby 'because, as people, they know-it-all, then you are failing them as caregivers. *As a minority group, we know that even in the medical field, it is taught that they (minority ethnic groups) have a high pain tolerance so they can bear pain longer.*

There is so much bias that comes with discrimination. Because, for many parts, it sits deep in the foundation of the systems, many either follow the rules without question, do not want to call it out, do not recognize it, or are playing oblivion. Discrimination is not a subject that is easy to solve where healthcare happens, but we can educate our folk on the importance of education and knowing what and when to be vocal about their wants, hopes, and needs.

Making real personal connections with others, not only remotely, but is also essential. Suppose you are near a mother/parent group. It is vital to avail yourself and creates your village.

Parenting can be very isolating and lonely. Sharing space with people who understand your journey can be refreshing, given that in such a space, there is no reason to justify your reasons or decisions with other parents who don't get you.

Nineteen

QUESTIONS TO ASK YOUR CARE PROVIDERS

Before your medical file gets closed and returned to the shelf, write down some questions.

Truth be told, the postpartum appointment at the hospitals has nothing to do with the mothers, mostly. When you think of the number of scans an expectant parent receives in the last trimester compared to the number of contacts they receive after, it's diabolic to even fathom why the need for their mental health is still taken lightly.

In current times where there is still a lot of concern for postpartum depression and WHO warning about speaking to parents about incidents like the shaken baby syndrome, one is left to be amazed at how little the birthing person really receives attention. The concern and focus are still on the baby and whether they are adding on weight and how their umbilical cord has dried and healed enough.

Unfortunately, the one focus for you as a newborn mother is:

(1) When you can think of trying to get pregnant again
(2) Contraception that you can use from now on

Many people were born artists as in they know how to slap the makeup so well that the thought for many care providers that woman who looks spanking good could never have postpartum issues or mental health issues. Some women complain they felt they were not heard at their appointments.

Many women complain about the disconnection that exists, especially in the western world where in many places including hospitals one is made to feel like they are a product being passed through a conveyer belt because of how detached the people who are supposed to care for them, worry for them and offer custom-support are very stiff, detached and seem rushed with time to complete a full clinic list in time that makes sense.

So for many of the couples who I have been privileged to support and share their life's experiences of becoming parents, I remind them to go ready with their question lists especially if they are under specialist care because most probably they would meet a whole team of Drs together, something that does not happen easily and therefore to take advantage of that opportunity and ask all questions and receive detailed answers.

1. What does today's appointment mean?
2. How did the birth go? Do they have anything to share, questions, etc.?
3. Did my child receive all their first or initial treatments like Vitamin K, etc.?
4. Am I being discharged from your care now? What happens when the file gets closed and a situation arises?

5. Can I still contact the midwife or do I now go back to my GP/general doctor's care?
6. Was there anything that happened during my birth that we should discuss for subsequent pregnancies?
7. Contraception advise and options available

Ask questions and ask them to elaborate further if they made little sense initially. Asking does not mean you are stupid, people ask to understand. If you have a valid reason to argue a case, do it respectfully because nothing comes out of being rude and uncooperative.

Twenty

FROM ONE PARENT TO ANOTHER - TIPS

Parenting / Mothering is supposed to be enjoyed and experienced as a learning opportunity for both parent and child, not something to be endured. Therefore, aim to thrive through your postpartum and not only survive it. Your postpartum period can be calm and tranquil with planning and often not a full bank account. Ancestrally, folk came from near and far bearing gifts to help with the health of mother and child and the community at large.

Not every Pregnancy and the postpartum period will be the same. **Enjoy and learn** from all the experiences you will have because every one of them will teach you something about yourself, your strength and your weakness, and the experience will test you. Try to stay grounded through it.

Plant the seeds of safety and availability with your children from the start. It is ok for them to still crawl into your bed at 14 if they need to and can for safety and trust. Not every child thrives with being separated from their parents. There is a reason you, as the parent, are what your child needs in their time of need. Do not tire or dismiss that.

Strength: You don't always have to be strong. Sometimes you would need to cuss, scream or have a good cry. It is ok to feel defeated and deflated sometimes. Remember, even the strongest people need others to cry and be weak, too. It will be ok. Pick yourself up, though, and continue. Don't stay in that position of feeling like a failure.

Accept that running yourself to the ground will help no one in your family. Your children need a parent who is able and capable of looking after them. Take your breaks and pause without guilt. Allow yourself the moment to drink a cup of tea whilst it is still hot or warm. Normalize taking a break without feeling like you have to run yourself to the ground. That is not what parenting is. The washing-up will still be there tomorrow, so create the time and accept that some things will have to wait and you cannot be everything and everyone to everyone.

Do not dwell so much on what happened last time. Try to enjoy your subsequent experience and learn from your previous experience, too. Your first experience does not have to be the only experience you will hold close and dear. Your first experience will inevitably make you a teacher of some sort to your friends' group because then you can share what it was like for you, for your family, how you dealt with xyz, and also give tips that may be beneficial to others. Look at the experience as a learning curve.

Believe in yourself and your decisions regarding the welfare of your baby and children. Doubt will always be present, but believe that you are doing the best for your children's needs and if they could speak or respond to you, they would.

Jealousy: Sibling jealousy is real. The best way I have found to have worked and received feedback also is by using the time when the baby is sleeping to do things with your older child. Involve them throughout the process, not just the belly part, but with life afterward. Ask for their opinion on things like rompers and choice of clothing for the day to keep the excitement of a sibling present. Many times your oldest child has not registered that the baby is at home to stay there now. There is still a void when visitors or family members leave your house. Many children wander in their minds. *Aren't you forgetting someone?* Or *when is this one going to be picked up?*'

Time: Try to create time with your children individually. Every one of them will have different needs and capabilities and therefore 1:1 attention and moments will go a long way. If you have other children or more than one child, create an agenda where you spend time with the children individually through activities or simply dates where you can find out how they are feeling, where they are struggling, and what can be done about it, are they happy? Why not and what can you do as a parent to ensure they are?

Answers: Many times we search for answers which are under our noses. Focus and learn the cues from your own baby and eventually your family's needs. Not one book will cover that for you.

Unsolicited advice: will pour unto you from all angles of the world. It is human to want to contribute sometimes, even without being asked for the contribution. There are many expectations and advice that come with new life. It is normal to get folk within your circle and those not (so basically unsolicited advice) from the moment you announce a pregnancy or the belly begins to show, and the moment they see you push a pram.

Let it go: If I can give you one tip? Nod and smile. Choose your battles. There will be so many times you would want to chew someone alive (haha, trust me on this one) but choose where you want to divert your energy. Your baby needs you in equilibrium with yourself. Do not spoil the moment because of someone's unsolicited comment that ruins your mood and shuts you down. Choose peace. Let it go.

Sleep when the baby sleeps is advice that does not apply to many, nor does it make sense. When the baby sleeps, parents catch up with everything that they are pending because the focus is on the baby when they are awake. Sleep when the baby is sleeping applies to parents with partners to share responsibilities.

Clean your ITS - (UnderPits, Tits, and the naughty bits too) Every moment you get! Because in the westernized setting of the postpartum period, you may not have the moment to really clean yourself after your day starts and for a few days, maybe. Start your days like you have a meeting every day. Take your shower, do your make-up if you do that regularly, dress up, and look human daily. By doing this, you make sure that you stay on top of things and that you do not fall into the resentful pit.

The beginning is hard for everyone; I was not exempt. As much as we would love to believe and hope deep within us, we would be like the content creators on Instagram who seem to have gotten it all together.. the reality is different. So don't fall for that. What you look at is an edited version that is used to portray only that part where the parents look so collected and together with the parenting that it makes you doubt yourself. The same advice I give to clients 'do not watch one born every minute whilst pregnant' is the same one I use in their postpartum, bleeding, pain, losing it, tears, sweat and lack of sleep are all part of the parenting game. Go with the flow and leave comparing-aunty outside your home, otherwise, you are in for a depressive start.

Social media and society have put so much weight on women and birthing people it feels overwhelming sometimes from the moment you test positive. Do not despair. The truth is; nobody is exempt from those early painful days when they cannot sit down comfortably because of tearing or simply bruising from childbirth. Few are exempt from the tears out of nowhere on the 4th or 5th day after childbirth. Few are exempt from getting mama-brain-freeze, where you had the memory so pitched up, and then you end up having post-it notes everywhere because suddenly your brain has become a sieve.

What is usually shown is **the last click** bearing the perfect parts where all the children are standing in line and staring at the camera, laughing or smiling the perfect way, where the make-up looks crisp, and where the babies are simply angels. What you should have at the back of your head is that these parents also shouted 'stand straight! Remove the fingers from your nose, Smile properly, Stop moving, and Don't speak...

The whole tirade of orders and frustrations followed that picture-perfect you stumbled on.

Nobody is born a mother: This is one area that many new parents struggle with because there is an expectation that you would feel maternal from the first glimpse of your baby's face.

Whilst that would be amazing, it is not guaranteed you would fall head-over-heels for your newborn baby. Remember, love grows, and sometimes that is a reality after the birth of the baby that the mother/birthing person needs time to build and then allow love to grow between themselves and their baby.

Feel it all: Postpartum flow of tears is very normal. It is as if the pieces of the birth even come together and then you realize what a badass you really were having birthed the whole baby! Don't shy from showing those emotions. It is very normal that this moment will come and you cannot explain why or what triggered you. It is the postpartum tears, and they are very normal.

Breastfeeding: although BEST is not so easy for many new parents. It is a craft you both have to learn, and patience and intentional support is the only thing that will help you both succeed with it.

Twenty-One

POSTPARTUM STORIES SHARED WITH ME

I asked intentionally if people wanted to share their experiences so that you, the reader, can take from their experiences to create your own or resonate and learn from their experiences. These women have attended my birth classes, I attended their births, and some of them have come into my weekly clubhouse rooms. Each experience shared may be shared here and please note that some names were changed to protect the sharers as they wished that.

One of my many postpartum mums (she/her) recently shared that:

' it took a lot of energy from me trying to justify my needs to stay in bed and be. Without needing to put a front, needing to be clapped for, for being active, up and running at day 3 after childbirth. When the whole clan came, and my body simply refused to get up, I knew I should not fight it. I knew it was not right, but we have normalized this kind of behavior around new parents that we praise them for being strong to a point that they fear being vulnerable with their own loved ones. There is nothing strong about running around still bleeding because folk will then clap for us and see our strength.

Strength is accepting that you have birthed a baby, need to rest, and the world needs to come to you to celebrate you. Strength admitting honestly, you need help. Strength is saying it is not a bed of roses, it is a learning experience, full of trial and error and welcoming those interested in experiencing it with you, to get dirty, get messy, get crazy, emotionally tired, get involved in the upbringing of that child, and honestly enjoy being a part of their lives.

Thank you, Naomie for writing this book. It is one that is so straightforward and needs to be in every home where pregnancy and babies have existed or are prophesied because this information, this knowledge, and this wisdom is like the nose in our faces. We simply don't see it.'

LISA & DAVID - *Parents of Milena (6 months old)*

I remember the day like yesterday, and feel very honored Naomie asked me if I was ok to share our story in this book to encourage others that the hard work is in planning the birth you envisage.

Communication is key, trusting that your team has an honest interest in helping you, staying open-minded to receive, and then education is the complete package you need. 9 months is really not enough to learn it all therefore get yourself a team that will help you see a little of what you aspire to achieve and even if it does not end up being how you thought it would for whatever reasons, you know in your heart that the people you had around you stood with you through it, and they would support you further.

I had just woken up as per usual, and David was in the kitchen making breakfast because I was getting slower in the mornings. My waters broke as I was talking to my belly in bed. Only 29 weeks was how long I was. I could not believe it at first. At first, I thought maybe I just peed myself, but I had no sensation.

I called up my local hospital, and I was advised to go in immediately. And that is how the breakfast before the birth of Milena happened. Suddenly, we were engulfed with questions between ourselves and our team.

We called up Naomie, who was our Doula, and she came straight to the hospital. She had a list of questions for us to ask our caregivers' team, which took a lot of weight off our backs because then we didn't have to think about what we would ask. Having a Doula helped in the sense that she gave tips sometimes individually, but she focused on my husband more because his mental awareness was active, unlike mine

I went through the stages of birth alert and was in control of the events. Naomie worked with my husband David to keep me hydrated and comfortable. Lots of stories were shared, lots of laughter, and silence when we all needed some calm. The whole atmosphere was just so ideal.

Naomie was quite known in this hospital, so it was easy for her to convey our aspirations for the birth we hoped to achieve. The whole team was for our benefit, and it gave me so much confidence because everybody was transparent and information was conveyed to be used when it was needed, and we were given the space to think and then respond.

I slept through it, and I remember from the evening we had had with Naomie for the preparation evenings, where she really prepared David with information and had us talk about our expectations in front of each other ahead of time. David knew what was expected of him. He looked at Naomie many times for confirmation, many times without words being exchanged between them because they had formed a bond and had discussed that they would strive to keep me in my bubble as much as they could, which is why it had to be her in the room with us.

I reached 9cms without so much anxiety or screaming. I was in control and had the right faces in front of me. Naomie would wipe my face with a wet flannel whenever I needed it and helped me sway left and right in silence and in words when I needed to hear her. Shortly after, the midwife arrived and asked where I wanted to birth, and where I felt ok to birth, and I birthed on all fours. Before long, I couldn't keep my legs on the floor without shaking. And I felt I needed to voice myself to achieve the last leg.

Well, up and behold... I birthed Milena on all fours after 5 pushes with David catching her before placing her on my chest. We had discussed the possibility of having postpartum support after our

Kraamzorg left and boy! We were glad we booked Naomie!! I don't want to advertise here but when you have someone caring for you in this phase, you cannot put enough price on it. You not having to think about food. Food is one aspect of the postpartum period and many find it a bigger puzzle to solve that it leaves some in a panic, almost. What she did was discuss our food allergies beforehand, the days she was going to come in 6 weeks after childbirth, and what we could expect when she came.

The support we had in that room was out of this world. If I can advise anyone, it is to iterate on the importance of getting support in any phase of your growth. Be it a class only focussing on the pregnancy, support at birth, or postpartum support because we were never meant to do any of it alone and it can get too much and overwhelming quickly.

Naomie cooked delicious meals. She is very in tune with her traditional ways, which we loved because what she does is wisdom passed down to her from her own lineage and birth line. With having her on board, I got massaged every time she came. I received a body wrap every time she came. I could speak to her easily and share my hardships with emotions and overwhelm, and she guided me in the most gentle way. It made my recovery very calm, without judgment but full of love and encouragement, and it left us resilient to face parenting as it presented itself.

If money is not an issue, book yourself the support you need because 8 or 10 days is not enough and sometimes family does not do a good job like someone you pay. If money is a problem, get a group of good friends or family that will support you at this moment and put in place plans, so that everyone knows what will be expected of them ahead of time

ANNEMARIE & THOMAS - *Full term stillborn birth*

Our experience was quite shocking, and it opened my eyes in a way that has been profound. Our baby Channel was born full term. I remember waking up to a pool of water I thought I had peed the bed. The patch was not urine. I called the midwife, and she said she would head to me. So we waited without worry or the slightest idea that this would be a miss. I just thought maybe I will go into labor earlier and we were ready to meet our little girl. The midwife came and tried to check for a heartbeat and at first; we thought she heard something but then confirmed she was only catching mine. She tried a few times again, and all she heard was my heartbeat.

She suggested calling the local hospital to see if they could do a scan there. She transferred us for further scanning. We arrived at the hospital within 20 minutes, and we were now worried because the triage nurse who received us was already informed, not sharing much, but we could see that she wanted to change their suspicions.

She took us into the room, offered a glass of water or tea and announced she would be back shortly. We settled into the room. Deep within, I was praying as I had never prayed before. I was panicking within myself and I could see my husband trying really hard to keep positive and offering me strength.

Then the nurse came back into the room and asked if she could scan my belly. We were ready because I wanted closure too that it is all well with our child. So she got everything ready and began scanning. She went silent at first, then when she spoke she said she was going to get a colleague to confirm something for her. The colleague walked in and they both nodded shortly after she also tried to scan me. They were also only hearing my heartbeat. Then it was confirmed that the baby's heartbeat could not be found. The room was spinning, and I wanted it to stop. I wanted so badly to wake up from the dream because I was not enjoying it anymore. It had turned into a terrible nightmare. I could not even bring myself to cry. I was in shock. HOW?

The nurses excused themselves shortly after saying some things that up to today; I do not recall what they said. The room was full of echoes, and they left us to digest what we were just told. We hugged in the room, and I wailed like an injured animal. I could not believe I heard what I did and I could not accept that was the news for us. WHY? I kept crying, and Thomas hugged me tighter, and we just cried together.

Later that evening, Thomas informed family and friends of our news, and some wanted to come immediately, but I was not in the mood to be around people. So we agreed they would be informed once the baby was born, so those who wanted to see her could come and see her and pay their last respects, too. That same evening another nurse came into the room and explained the procedure, and that I would be given a pill to help birth our baby if contractions did not start immediately they broke my waters tomorrow because live babies help with the birth, and it can be hard for a baby who is no longer alive to help you with the process.

So we had the evening to cry, pray for our little girl together and decide if we wanted our doula present the following day. Naomie was our birth doula, turned bereavement doula and she offered us space where we needed it but also helped us prepare questions we could ask and gave tips on how we could personalize our experience too.

We were happy we had booked a full spectrum doula because nobody speaks about the possibility of finding yourselves at this moment when the baby does not get home. With the birth preparation sessions we had with Naomie, she touched on Plan B ahead of time, so facing it was manageable because it was not so new a topic. Talking about it beforehand helps because it brings an understanding that a healthy baby is not a guarantee.

Naomie agreed to change our birth plan when she went home that evening, to resonate with what we wanted now with our news, etc. We were still going to get some hand and feet prints if possible. Then she helped plan the moments after with the nurses within the unit where we were admitted. After all the planning, we bid her goodbye, and we were to see Naomie the following day.

The following day, Naomie returned with something in her arms. She was making a blanket gift for our Channel which was very thoughtful. She also had made two knitted hearts, one that would go with the baby and one that would remain with us. Her preparation was very humbling because until she arrived, we only saw sadness and heartache. With her permission, we used the blanket she had made especially for Channel to cover her cot and also for the planned ceremony.

***JUDITH & KALAMA** - Ancestral Sacred RITES Postpartum experience*

When we found out we were expecting our baby, we were engulfed by every emotion you can think of. 9 months sounded far then, but really it went by fast. If I can encourage any new parents out there, it is to enjoy your pregnancy with all that comes with it. Sometimes there will be hurdles thought the journey, but the day you will hold your baby in your arms and feel their little chest move on your shoulders, you will see it really is worth it.

For Kalama and me, we knew we wanted to go back to ancestral times when not everything was researched and categorized as the bible truth. I spoke with my mother back in Zambia at length about how the postpartum period is handled, and she was thrilled that we were looking to go back to our roots. When we told her we had found a postpartum doula with ancestral wisdom, my mother was ecstatic.

The reason for us wanting to go back to ancestral wisdom was because of the gentle, holistic approach, which is very much needed in the moments following the birth of a baby. I couldn't imagine myself being coached to parent my child or being confused about what the book said and what another 'professional' person was also saying to me. I wanted to do things calmly with reason and understanding why that was.

Haste has no place where babies are concerned or newborn mothers at all. I remember saying to K how excited I was that we were blessed with a little one and how I look forward to doing xyz. I read books and thought in my head that I was prepared enough, but a good deal missed something; **the ancestral** knowledge. Many times when I had my midwife appointments, I felt a sense of disconnection from the old ways of doing things and sticking rigidly to evidence-based and if it had never been researched; it was not something to ask a medical person.

So we booked a postpartum doula ahead of time because a birth doula was not allowed during the pandemic. After the kraamzorg was finished on day 8, our postpartum doula arrived to continue with the care. What she offered was customized care and attention for the whole family. She focused on my mental health, allowing me the space to vent, learn and share without judgment, and felt heard. She checked in with us every other day, and we knew we could contact her whenever we had questions or something to share before she came by again.

She arrived with a plan at every appointment, and we knew beforehand what we needed to do to prepare the house ahead of time. Anyway, the 6 weeks went by fast, and even after all the love and care we had received, it still felt like she should have stayed longer. I began to understand what they mean back home 'The postpartum period is never 6-8 weeks, but eternal'. I felt I needed to be mothered even after the care of weeks.

I felt I needed someone to be there for me if I had questions. I felt I needed another parent I could call to share my frustrations with, to share my wins, and also exchange notes with. The beauty of the tribe became so clear, and I began to yearn for childbearing years back home where everyone was available to you and your baby for all eternity.

It hit me then that surely the old ways are new ways. We should go back in time and embrace the gentle, caring, nurturing ways of mothering mothers. Of pulling together in celebrations of both life and death. To always have a village behind you where your well-being was everyone's interest, and your family's growth and children's life was everyone's responsibility. Where a person was regarded as a parent, whether they carried or birthed them. Boundaries are created without status. There is an automatic ancestral knowledge in understanding of the need for support in these early and eternal fragile moments.

SHARONDA NEVELS: Ancestral Postpartum Wisdom

Sharonda is a virtual friend who attends my clubhouse rooms weekly when I host them. This is her story.

When I had my baby, things were going on around me. I had no control over it. I knew I was dealing with postpartum depression, but I was not due for my 6-week checkup after the baby until 2 more weeks. So, I didn't come out of my room.

My appetite was nonexistent. Food or eating didn't come to mind first. I would not sleep. I was scared my baby would stop breathing during the night. It was awful! My mother came and got me out of the room one day, and I made it to the bonus room.

That was the start. And then she told me, 'I think you have baby blues. I replied to her, 'no mama, I will not kill my baby, that is how the media portrays PPD/PPA. My doctor couldn't work me in to see him. It is February at this point, my mother said 'You know what? go hug a tree and play with some dirt. I thought she had lost it!! Was she going senile? But she took my baby and led me to the tree. I started playing with the bark of the tree, the leaves, the little insects because it was a little warm for February that year.

She left me outside and would not let me inside the house. I called it 'house arrest'. When I had my babies, I have gone back home to her for 3 months. When you are there for postpartum care, she takes care of the baby and she will even make food, so no fast food. At night, she would take the baby whilst you slept and she would bring the baby to you when the baby was hungry. I absolutely thank her for her sacrifice in her older age to have come forth to care, nurture and love on me

Twenty-Two

HOMEMADE RECIPES TO TRY

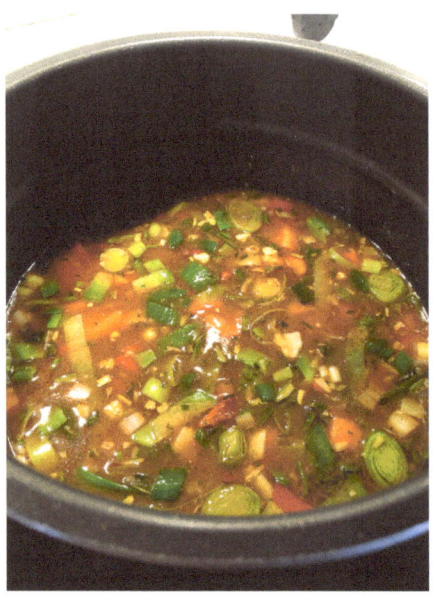

Wholesome Meatballs Soup
Naomie Karma

This is one of my signature soups because of how tasty, easy to make and simply wholesome it is. It is so filling you may not even need to eat it with anything, depending on your appetite of course . I love that you can make it with or without meat for a vegetarian version

Ingredients:

Meatballs

1. 1 Leek - washed and sliced
2. 1 Red onion - diced
3. 2 chopped tomatoes
4. 3/4 Carrots - peeled, cleaned and sliced
5. 1 Courgette/Zucchini
6. 3 tablespoons Olive Oil
7. 1 stock cube
8. 2/3 potatoes - depending on size
9. water - add until you get the taste and consistency you like
10.

Method:

1. In a pot put your Olive oil
2. Add your diced red onion. Cook until thawed
3. Add tomatoes and cook until soft
4. Add your meatballs and brown. Then cover to cook softly
5. Then add your carrots, Stock cube and some water and cover to cook
6. Then add the soft vegetables, Courgette and Leek
7. Add your potatoes - diced
8. Add some more water if still salty and if diluted enough leave as is
9. Reduce heat and let is simmer for about 10 minutes
10. Serve hot/warm

PUMPKIN SOUP

Pumpkin Soup is one of y favorite soups because of how tasty and easy it to make. The ingredients are not overwhelming either. It keeps really well in the fridge and freezes well too. It is warming and filling at the same time. In your postpartum period, Pumpkins are known to be nutritious in that they are full of magnesium, folate, iron, vitamin B - 6 and Phosphorus which help with reducing sleeplessness and improves energy

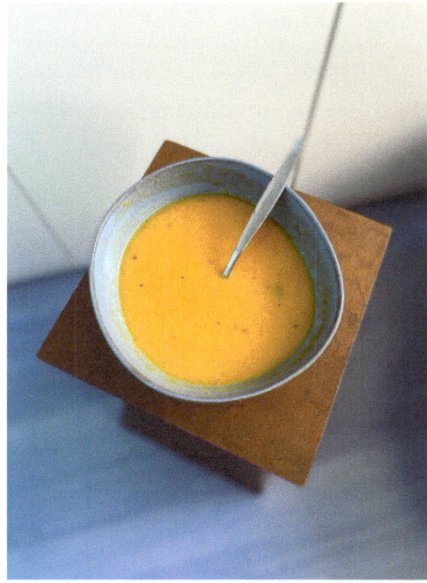

Pumpkin Soup
Naomie Karemi

Ingredients

1. 1 big carrot
2. An apple - that you can cook
3. A pumpkin
4. 2 stock cubes
5. 1 small ginger stem
6. 1 orange
7. 1 red onion
8. 1 clove of ginger

Method:

1. Wash and cut your vegetable is small cubes
2. In a pot add a little bit of Olive oil or Coconut oil
3. Add your diced red onion
4. Then add your pieces of Pumpkin and cook for a bout 10 minutes

5. Add your carrots and cook for another 10 minutes
6. Then add your potatoes, the mix of ginger, garlic and stock cubes
7. Add some water to cook everything and cover to cook until soft
8. Reduce heat and leave it to simmer for 5 minutes
9. Add your pressed Orange juice from the orange - check out for seeds before adding
10. Stir gently for a little bit
11. Let it rest for a few minutes
12. With a hand mixer, blend everything until smooth
13. To add a little bit of smoothness, add coconut cream whilst it is still hot and mix thoroughly
14. Serve warm with toasted slices of bread and sprinkle some roasted pumpkin seeds on top

OVEN BAKED / AIR FRIED CHICKEN WITH ALL TRIMMINGS

I love oven dishes for what they provide. Considering you can whip this one in one pot, the flavors of everything mixed will leave you wowed. It is a healthy dish but always brings a feast to it. It's in the need for everything to cook a certain way and then come together that makes this dish a winner even in my own house. If i can get my children to eat vegetables? It is through this dish

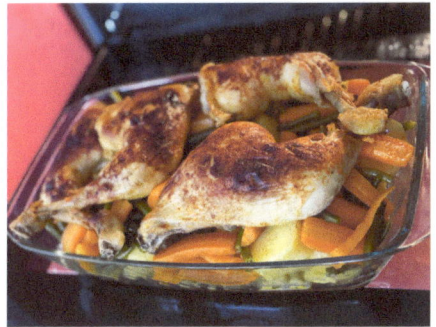

Oven baked/ Air fried Chicken with trimmings

Ingredients

1. Chicken (full or legs)
2. I bag potatoes
3. 5/6 carrots
4. 1 bag green beans
5. Any other vegetables of your choice like Peas or Ben maize on a cob
6. Gravy

Method:

1. In the airfryer out your chicken and let it cook till brown and cooked inside
2. In a pot steam your potatoes until soft but not cooked through
3. Steam carrots, green beans and then add everything to one big tray or the air fryer

You could even cook everything individually and then mix it all in an oven dish If cooking the chicken in a slow cooker first, be sure to cook it on the preset button (poultry) for half the time set, otherwise it will over cook the chicken. Once cooked through add it to your already precooked potatoes, steamed vegetables and let the tray sit in the oven for a while while you make the gravy

Gravy

1. In another pot add your gravy granules and some warm water first
2. Once fully mixed without lumps bring to the boil
3. Start slowly then add the heat
4. Whisk or mix as it warms up to avoid it lumping on the bottom of the pan
5. If too thick add water. If too think in a separate bowl, mix gravy granules, mix then pour mixture in the pot already cooking
6. Mix until you get the consistency you like
7. Pour a little bit of it on to the potatoe and chicken mix
8. Leave some aside to serve with
9. Serve it warm and enjoy!

LOADED QUICHE

The benefit of a Quiche is how versatile it is as a dish. You can almost never go wrong with this one. It freezes really well meaning it will always be ready for you to eat and it remains scrumptious when defrosted too. You do not even need to go extravagant with a Quiche which calls for you to use everything vegetable that you already have in the fridge. It fills you up so well too, accompanied with a cup of light soup or a side salad

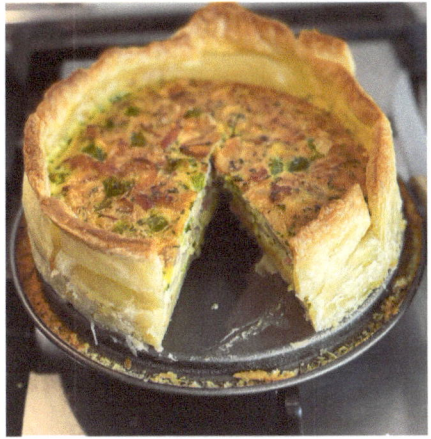

Loaded Quiche
Naomie Karemi

Ingredients

1. Everything in your freezer
2. 1 Medium sized round baking tin
3. 1 bag of potatoes
4. 1 Leek
5. 1 pack of baking pastry
6. 1 small pack of cooking cream
7. 3 eggs
8. Meat if you have any
9. Salt or stock cube
10. Butter to spread in the tin
11. Shredded cheese

Method:

1. Peel your potatoes, cut, wash and have them ready
2. In a pan boil your potatoes
3. Put your greens in another pan, a stock cube for taste on low heat, not to cook

4. Prepare your baking tin
5. Smear some butter around and at the base
6. Lay the tin with your pastry sheets
7. Then fork the pastry sheets inside the baking tin to allow for heat to bake through
8. Check your potatoes are nicely ready, not too cooked
9. Add Potatoes, all your greens, eggs, salt, and mix thoroughly.
10. If dry, mix a small amount of cooking cream to add fluid
11. Pour your mix inside the baking tin
12. Top up with shredded cheese
13. Bake in the middle shelf of the oven at 200 degrees and for 20 minutes.
14. Check with a fork to make sure the inside is cooked and not sticky. If it is sticky, you can add 5 minutes
15. Then switch the oven off and allow the Quiche to cook with the heat only
16. When satisfied, remove from the oven
17. Allow to rest and then remove from the baking tin
18. Serve warm with a salad on the side, a cup of soup or as it is
19. It freezes really good. If freezing, best done on the day it was made/cooked

FLUFFY PANCAKES

Ingredients

1. 1 cup of flour
2. 1 cup of milk
3. 1 spoonful of baking powder
4. A pinch of salt
5. Pinch of sugar

6. Cinnamon (optional)
7. Desiccated coconut (optional)
8. 1 egg..

Method:

1. Mix the dry ingredients separately... Then add them to your 'wet ingredients' and mix them well... A hand mixer should do the job coz you don't want lumps left right and centre.
2. Heat your pan and add some butter, I prefer this because it melts and your pancakes won't be too oily (some use cooking oil but I don't like the taste).
3. Once the pan is heated up, reduce the heat to medium-low and pour your batter (mixture) right in the middle and allow it to spread.
4. The quality of the pan also matters. A flat non-stick pan is perfect.
5. Do not flip it until some air spaces/bubbles have formed on the side facing you..

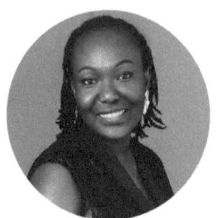

Naomie Karemi is a native Kenyan/British citizen living in the Netherlands. With her Dutch husband, Tom, they are raising three amazing children. One of their children is living with a disability from a birth incident and genetic variation, but as a couple, they have stood taller with and for each other in raising him. Naomie is a born leader, a firstborn in a family of five (3 children and both parents) and therefore, decision-making and leading is a virtue that is instilled in her already. In many of her work, with groups of friends, she takes on the role of the listener and adviser alike

Naomie calls herself the 4th generation Traditional Birth worker because her female lineage, starting from her maternal grandmother, has served in the realm of Birth and Postpartum work. Her maternal grandmother was a traditional Midwife back in her village, assisting in many births, including those of Naomie's cousins. Naomie was the grandchild who was welcomed to witness childbirth and introduced to being of service to new mothers after childbirth, one being her youngest Aunt following the birth of her cousin. From a young age, the excitement of being in a space with new life and family adjustments has been imprinted in her. She was given tasks like being sent back then to boil water and get the razor, making sure it was still closed (sterile) in readiness for the birth of a baby.

She is currently a certified Birth and Bereavement Doula. She studying for her Dutch Diploma in Maternity Nursing, hoping to work more in the holistic way of mothering mothers and their families later on. Her work covers the whole realm of Birth, Postpartum and Bereavement support too.

Therefore, it is no wonder that she shares ancestral wisdom in this aspect of Postpartum, the importance of family and support